This book tackles the complex and oft[e] ived experience of mid-life, with insights fro[m] dred women. In these pages, the reader is in[v] [st]ories, challenging the invisibility often associ[ated] [ult]ately drawing us towards a collective reimagin[ing].

— **Molly Andrews**, co-director, Association for Narrative Research and Practice

If you're a woman facing the beautiful, messy, occasionally harsh realities of mid-life, this book is for you. It offers a candid exploration of what it means to be a middle-aged woman in modern western society, a role which sees us at once indispensable and ignored. It's an eye-opening read.

— **Catherine Clark**, co-founder, The Honest Talk

This is the midlife book we've been missing! Ann Douglas demystifies midlife and launches a conversation with inclusion, justice, compassion and honesty at its core. Navigating the Messy Middle will be well-loved, dogeared, underlined, and passed from friend to friend. It will encourage continued conversations between women who, after reading this book, will know for sure that they aren't alone.

— **Sara Smeaton**, midlife coach

In this comprehensive overview of mid-life, Ann Douglas weaves a powerful tapestry of narratives, rich with the colours of many voices. The result is a precious gift for women feeling lost, desperate or alone in midlife, since Douglas reveals, vibrantly, how peril is outweighed by potential, and that midlife can be a "journey of becoming." This is an important and much-needed book.

— **Beth Powning**, author of Edge Seasons: A Midlife Year

The best thing about Ann Douglas's perspective, as always, is her understanding that one-size-fits-all advice fits no one. Instead, in Navigating the Messy Middle, readers will discover an empowering guide to finding one's own way through the ups and downs of midlife, a time when seeking strength in connection, embracing the changeability of the physical self, and focusing on one's real values and priorities can create a powerful moment of (finally!) becoming.

— **Kerry Clare**, author of Waiting for a Star to Fall

If we're lucky, we all occasionally have one of those evenings with friends where we vent about everything rattling around in our brains and lives, and realize that the answer to the question "Is it just me?" is a resounding no. This book is one of those evenings between two covers, delivered with Douglas's signature wisdom, perspective, warmth and wit.

— **Shannon Proudfoot**, former Ottawa bureau chief, Maclean's

In *Navigating the Messy Middle*, Ann Douglas gives us the context, the compassion and the courage needed to understand the challenges, gifts and opportunities that midlife presents. It reads like both a manifesto and a heart-to-heart with your closest friends.

— **Brandie Weikle**, editor and publisher, *The New Family*

Our culture paints a vague yet bleak picture of menopause, and the result is a population of women who see their first hot flash as the beginning of the end. But midlife is about more than menopause. It's nuanced and multifaceted, and where there can sometimes be misery, there can also be magic, as Ann Douglas illustrates persuasively in her new book, *Navigating the Messy Middle*. Written clearly and compellingly with a mix of science-backed information and real-life stories, *Navigating the Messy Middle* will inevitably find a wide, appreciative audience. Reading it made me feel seen, understood and empowered, and my anxiety about this period in my life has been replaced by curiosity and optimism. If you buy one book about midlife, make it this one.

— **Kim Shiffman**, editor-in-chief, *Today's Parent*

Applying surgical myth-busting to harmful narratives that disappear middle-aged women, Ann Douglas takes us on a life-affirming journey. Reading it has been a bit of an emotional journey. I think most women will have the same reaction—feeling seen, validated and celebrated!

— **Kelly Carmichael**, former executive director, Fair Vote Canada

I have appreciated Ann Douglas' insights on parenting for many years. She is kind, honest and clear-eyed, and much less patronizing than other relationships writers. She puts these skills to great use in *Navigating the Messy Middle*, which comes at a perfect time for me as I try to evolve into the next stage of my life. This book shows middle-aged women that we're not alone, while encouraging us to prioritize what makes our unique selves satisfied and happy.

— **Denise Balkissoon**, Ontario bureau chief, *The Narwhal*
and former executive editor, *Chatelaine*

In *Navigating the Messy Middle*, Ann Douglas challenges the prevailing narrative that women in midlife are a product past their prime. Combatting this culturally prescribed march toward invisibility, Douglas centres a diversity of women who, through sharing their stories, weave a broader, kinder, more accurate and more inclusive narrative that is ripe with the realities, possibilities, complexities and contradictions experienced by women in midlife.

— **Kathryn Adams-Sloan**, chair of the Women's Caucus to the
Canadian Association for Social Work Education

Navigating the Messy Middle

A Fiercely Honest and Wildly Encouraging Guide for Midlife Women

— ANN DOUGLAS —

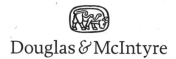

Douglas & McIntyre

Douglas and McIntyre (2013) Ltd.
P.O. Box 219, Madeira Park, BC, VON 2H0
www.douglas-mcintyre.com

Edited by Caroline Skelton
Indexed by Ellen Hawman
Cover design by Naomi MacDougall
Text design by Libris Simas Ferraz / Onça Publishing
Printed and bound in Canada
Printed on stock made from 100% recycled fibres

 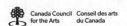 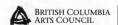

Douglas and McIntyre acknowledges the support of the Canada Council for the Arts,
the Government of Canada and the Province of British Columbia through the BC
Arts Council.

Library and Archives Canada Cataloguing in Publication
Title: Navigating the messy middle : a fiercely honest and wildly encouraging guide
    for midlife women / Ann Douglas.
Names: Douglas, Ann, 1963- author.
Description: Includes index.
Identifiers: Canadiana (print) 20220233268 | Canadiana (ebook) 20220233276 |
    ISBN 9781771623438 (softcover) | ISBN 9781771623445 (EPUB)
Subjects: LCSH: Middle-aged women—Life skills guides. | LCSH: Middle age—
    Psychological aspects. | LCSH: Middle age—Social aspects. |
    LCSH: Middle-aged women.
Classification: LCC HQ1059.5 .D68 2022 | DDC 305.244/2–dc23

To Janet, Lorna and Sandra,
sisters extraordinaire and
fellow midlife travellers

Stories bring together the reconstructed past and the imagined future, and provide messy human lives with some semblance of meaning, order, and purpose.

— **Dan P. McAdams**, "The Life Narrative at Midlife"

The stories we compose are our only map.

— **Sara Lawrence-Lightfoot**, *The Third Chapter: Passion, Risk, and Adventure in the 25 Years After 50*

We're only here for a minute. We're here for a little window. And to use that time to catch and share shards of light and laughter and grace seems to me the great story.

— **Brian Doyle**, *One Long River of Song: Notes on Wonder*

Table of Contents

Part III Soul: On Navigating Change and Finding Community

Author's Note

Land acknowledgement

This book was written on the unceded ancestral territory of the Anishinaabeg people, people who have been living on and caring for this land since time immemorial. I am grateful for the opportunity to live and work in this beautiful place of lakes and trees, and to continue on my own journey of reconciliation. The best way I know how to live that journey is by supporting the LANDBACK movement, both locally and around the world. For me, this means encouraging other settlers to learn about this movement and to donate to Indigenous-led groups through the Nii'kinaaganaa Foundation's Pay Your Rent initiative, and to watch *Canada, It's Time for Land Back* with Pam Palmater, a six-minute video that has the potential to change your life and our world.

About the stories in this book

The stories in this book are based on detailed conversations and/or correspondence with the women who were interviewed for this book. In all cases, permission was obtained to quote these women and to share their experiences. In some situations, identifying details were changed to protect the privacy of the individuals involved. In other cases, pseudonyms were provided at the woman's request. I have edited and paraphrased some comments in the interests of clarity, while still striving to honour the spirit and intention of the original comments.

Medical disclaimer

This book is designed to provide you with general information about midlife development and health. This book is not intended to provide a complete or exhaustive treatment of this subject; nor is it a substitute for advice from the health practitioners who know you best. Seek medical attention promptly for any medical or psychological concern you may be experiencing. Do not take any medication without obtaining medical advice. All efforts were made to ensure the accuracy of the information contained in this publication as of the date of writing. The author and the publisher expressly disclaim any responsibility for any adverse effects arising from the use or application of the contents herein. While the parties believe that the contents of this publication are accurate, a licensed medical practitioner should be consulted in the event that medical advice is desired. The information contained in this book does not constitute a recommendation or endorsement with respect to any company or product.

Introduction

Midlife not quite what you expected?

Hey, join the club.

Most of us find ourselves being caught more than a little off guard, either by the way midlife is playing out or by the fact that it's happening at all.

Our youth-worshipping culture (and by that I mean mainstream Western culture) encourages us to deny the fact that we're actually growing older until the fact of our aging becomes completely undeniable, at which point we're encouraged to see it as either completely magical or totally miserable.

What we eventually figure out for ourselves is that it's actually a little of both—that the truth is somewhere in the middle: the messy middle.

I don't know about you, but I've reached a point in my life where I've come to celebrate that kind of messiness. It feels so much more honest than pretending that life is orderly or predictable, because it's not. Midlife is messy because life is messy. And simplistic narratives that try to pretend otherwise only serve to make an already tough life stage even harder. They leave us feeling woefully inadequate, convinced that we're doing midlife wrong.

We deserve so much better—midlife narratives that embrace rather than shy away from the messiness, stories that leave us feeling seen and celebrated as opposed to held to an impossibly high standard or (worse!) completely erased.

If you've read any of my earlier books, you won't be surprised to discover that conversations with other women are at the heart of this book.

In fact, they *are* the book.

I knew that if I wanted to do justice to a book like this, I needed to get inside the heads of a whole bunch of different women (and by that I mean any queer, non-binary, two-spirit, transgender or cisgender person who identifies as, or feels some affinity with, the role of "woman" as defined in Western culture right now). Sure, I'm a woman at midlife, but I'm only *one* woman at midlife—and a relatively privileged one at that. (I'm a white,* married, middle-class mother whose partner is a man.)

And so, from the moment I started researching this book, I made a point of deliberately seeking out the stories of women whose lives and experiences have been very different from my own, for reasons related to race, class, gender identity, sexual orientation, disability and more. I wanted to ensure that every woman who happens to pick up a copy of this book is able to see herself in at least some of the stories.

And that's the approach I chose to take as I started booking interviews: making phone calls, sending emails and scheduling Zoom meetings (because I was researching this book during the pandemic, pretty much everything was happening via Zoom). I approached everyone from friends to friends of friends to random strangers—people who didn't owe me a cup of coffee, let alone the time of day. And, overwhelmingly, these women said yes to my interview

---

* You'll note that when I write about whiteness or being white, I've chosen to use a lower-case letter in the word "white." This is the approach taken by Mona Eltahawy, Nikole Hannah-Jones, Ijeoma Oluo, Nora Loreto, Jessie Daniels and other writers whose work has had a huge impact on my own thinking, so I've made a conscious decision to follow their lead here.

requests. Maybe they were lonely. Maybe they were deeply craving human connection during a strange and uncertain time. Or maybe they simply welcomed the opportunity to reflect on their own unique journeys through midlife.

While I'll never know for certain what it was that led these women (well over one hundred of them) to trust me with their stories, I will be forever grateful. Not only did these conversations provide structure and meaning in my life at a time when I was feeling anxious and untethered, but they also renewed my faith in the essential goodness of other humans. You see, what I hadn't anticipated was just how honest and vulnerable the women I was interviewing would be willing to be—they trusted me with their hard-won wisdom because they wanted to make life better for some other woman, some future reader of this book who might be struggling in some sort of similar way. These women shared intimate details of their lives in a way that left me feeling awed by their frankness and their courage. They told me things about themselves that they hadn't dared to tell anyone else. I think you'll be deeply moved by their honesty and their bravery. I know I was. And I learned so much.

Midlife requires a radical imagination: a willingness to tell ourselves new and better stories about our lives.

We need stories that reject all the life-limiting narratives that only serve to make life harder and that actively conspire to rob us of joy.

We need stories that embrace—rather than erase—the nuance and contradiction that are woven into the very fabric of this life stage. We need stories that allow us to find meaning in all that messiness. And, above all, we need stories that remind us that we don't have to journey through this stage—or any stage of life—on our own.

We have the power to imagine these kinds of new and better stories into being—both for ourselves and with other women. And this kind of storytelling can be a powerful tool for making change. The mere act of telling a story to another person forces you to structure that story in a way that gives it meaning. And in creating that meaning for others, you end up unlocking that sense of meaning for yourself.

And that's when things start to get really exciting: in those moments of shared imagining. My story stops being just about me. Your story stops being just about you. Our stories start being about who we are—and who we aspire to be—together.

There's radical potential in that shared act of reimagining—from a chorus of women's voices rising together. As narrative psychologist Molly Andrews notes in her book *Narrative Imagination and Everyday Life*, "Imagination is not innocent, fuzzy and warm. Imaginative understanding can lead us to question the very foundations on which we have built order in our lives."

We can build new worlds on the foundations of those stories.

This is why this book is so rich in stories—why my entire life has been about telling stories, in fact. Because stories can change the world.

As feminist gerontologist Martha Holstein writes in her book *Women in Late Life: Critical Perspectives on Gender and Age*, "The model of women coming together to talk to one another and create transformational narratives can still be a powerful tool for change. Second-wave feminism demonstrated that when ideas radiate outward, political change can occur."

It's pretty clear to me that what we need right now is nothing short of transformational change—a radical reimagining of so many things, including what it means to be a woman at midlife. As Susan J. Douglas notes in her book *In Our Prime: How Older Women Are*

Reinventing the Road Ahead, "It's time not for a personal makeover, but for a cultural one."

The book you're holding in your hands is both a midlife love letter and a midlife lament, a book that both celebrates the beauty *and* rages at the many injustices of this life stage.

It also happens to be a book that is very much a product of the times in which it was written.

My agent negotiated the deal for this book in February 2020, just as the pandemic was beginning to be felt here in North America. The days and months that followed ended up changing everything, including me. I found myself launched into a multi-year journey into rethinking pretty much everything about my life. And judging by the depth of the conversations I was having with other women, I know I'm not the only one who was profoundly affected by this multi-layered experience of pause–the pandemic pause layered on top of the self-reflective pause that is so characteristic of midlife.

I wrote this book for those women.

I wrote this book for every caring, thinking woman who has ever been brave enough to ask herself the tough questions, who refuses to settle for things as they are, choosing instead to dare to imagine how things could be.

Who knows? Maybe I wrote this book for you.

— PART I —

Mind

The Thinking Part of Midlife

CHAPTER 1

Hello, Midlife?

Midlife managed to sneak up on me.

It wasn't until I started making plans to celebrate my fiftieth birthday that I finally recognized what was going on—where I *actually* was on my life journey. Not only had I arrived at midlife, but I'd been here for a while. I'd been sleepwalking through this life stage for the better part of a decade.

In fairness to my younger midlife self, I'd been sleepwalking for good reason. The early part of my midlife experience can best be described as a hurricane of converging storms: family emergencies, career curveballs and my own mental health crisis. I didn't have time to pause long enough to consider the bigger picture. I barely had time to breathe.

I haven't had just one midlife experience. I've actually had three.

The first part of my midlife story takes place around the time I was about to turn forty, a painful chapter in my life when I found myself reeling from the sudden and unexpected death of my mother. I was not only dealing with wave upon wave of complicated grief (I was also dealing with the fallout from some earlier traumas, including the equally sudden and unexpected stillbirth of my baby just a few years earlier) but also trying to meet the needs of four young children, each of whom was struggling in their own way; to deal with a series of nasty career-related curveballs; and to wrap my head around a recent bipolar disorder diagnosis. It was a lot to deal with. Too much, in fact. We're talking about a recipe for a very unhappy person, a depressed and anxious person who was rapidly approaching the point of burnout.

The second story picks up where the first story ends: in the Land of Burnout, with things completely falling apart. I remember feeling like I'd fallen into a black hole—a hole that was deep and dark enough that I was never going to be able to find my way out—a pretty terrible way to be feeling when you're only in your mid-forties. I missed a couple of critical work-related deadlines that threatened to jeopardize my entire career as an author. My physical and mental health hit rock bottom. My marriage was in only marginally better shape. I felt like I was treading water and like I was about to be swept under by a tidal wave of guilt—guilt for letting so many people down at the same time. It was exhausting just being alive.

And that brings us to the third and final story, the point in the trilogy at which things start to turn around. I managed to tap into support from a whole bunch of different people and to eventually find my way to a much happier, healthier place. That's not to say that everything in my life was suddenly perfect. This is real life, not fiction, after all. There were still some significant challenges waiting around the bend (hello, Meniere's disease; hello, house fire; hello, pandemic), but, as I headed into my fifties, I felt like I'd managed to figure some important things out. I'd learned some strategies for weathering the rough days and I'd come to recognize the importance of savouring the good days—plus I'd figured out how to spot the understated beauty in the days that fall somewhere in between. So while it's not quite a "happily ever after," it's a nice place to wrap up the trilogy, with me embracing my gloriously imperfect life and feeling cautiously optimistic about the future (which is pretty much where I find myself today).

Given how messy and complicated my own midlife experiences have been, I'm not about to settle for pat solutions or one-size-fits-all advice. Not for myself and certainly not for anyone else, including you! That's why, in researching and writing this book about midlife, I felt the need to go down so many different research rabbit holes in my quest for answers, and why I gravitated toward research that acknowledges what a complicated life stage this can be. It's also why self-knowledge, self-acceptance and self-compassion are such key threads in this book—because they made such a difference for me.

Midlife research roundup

It's hard to imagine a life stage that's more misunderstood than midlife—or about which there is more misinformation. Not only is there no road map, but you should consider yourself lucky if you actually manage to spot a road sign announcing that you've arrived in the territory. (Believe it or not, there isn't even a solid consensus around that!) It's a confusing life stage to live through and it's a confusing life stage to write about, which is why I ended up spending so much time researching this book, reading approximately a hundred books and poring through roughly a thousand journal articles on an eclectic mix of topics—everything from human development to narrative psychology to sociology.

I quickly discovered that even the most simple and straightforward questions don't necessarily yield simple or straightforward answers. Not when it comes to midlife! Sure, we may have endured roughly a half-century of media stories about the inevitability of the so-called midlife crisis, but as for actual scientific research about the life stage that is middle adulthood? That's still a relatively recent phenomenon. It wasn't until the mid-1990s that researchers actually got serious about studying midlife—practically a full century after the word "midlife" first found its way into a mainstream dictionary (the Funk & Wagnalls dictionary, in 1895, just in case you're wondering).

And even now, a couple of decades later, there's still a lot that we don't know about the lives of midlife adults. Even the simple question of timing is up for debate. While respected midlife researchers Frank J. Infurna, Denis Gerstorf and Margie E. Lachman define midlife as the years between forty and sixty, "plus or minus ten years," they also acknowledge that ordinary people (as opposed to midlife scholars) tend to narrow that range down a little—to the years between forty-four and fifty-nine. And in a much-cited article in the psychological journal *Research in Human Development*, Lachman noted that chronological age isn't necessarily the most helpful factor in deciding whether you've actually arrived at midlife. In other words, rather than narrowly fixating on the number of candles on your birthday cake, you'd be better off paying attention to major life transitions: having a kid leave home, experiencing the death of a parent or grappling with a mid-career shakeup at work.

Midlife is experiencing a bit of a shakeup of its own, by the way—one that has far-reaching implications for the current generation of midlife adults. Infurna, Gerstorf and Lachman have noted the combined impact of growing financial pressures, a shrinking social safety net and increased mental and physical health challenges in particular. To put it bluntly, this is not your parents' or grandparents' midlife experience. It's a whole lot messier and more precarious.

And that brings up another really important point: there's no such thing as a one-size-fits-all midlife experience. As Ashton Applewhite points out in her book *This Chair Rocks: A Manifesto Against Ageism*, "The longer we live, as more experiences inform our uniqueness, the more *different* from one another we become." And the more different our subsequent experiences end up being too. Those differences accrue over time in ways that can amplify inequality or privilege: there is as much as a twelve-year difference in life expectancy between those who are most and least well off. And that's just talking income. We also need to consider what journalist and activist Mona Eltahawy describes as "the Venn diagrams of oppression that color your life."

The challenge, of course, is in trying to unearth data that adequately captures the glorious diversity of midlife women. As I quickly discovered, much of the research tends to be centred on a very specific kind of midlife woman: a white, cisgender, married, middle-class woman with children. In other words, someone a lot like me. If you happen to go looking for research that takes a more intersectional approach to the lives of midlife women, well, you're going be looking pretty long and hard. Research that acknowledges that midlife isn't experienced in the same way by all women and that social and political identities such as race, class, gender, sexual identity and age intersect with one another in a way that amplifies both inequality and privilege—a concept developed and articulated by Kimberlé Crenshaw and other brilliant Black woman authors and scholars—continues to be as rare as a unicorn.

The good news is that there are some really groundbreaking and important books being written, books that look at women's lives through a much more intersectional lens. I have been particularly inspired by the work of Eltahawy, whose recent book, *The Seven Necessary Sins for Women and Girls*, highlights the urgent need to "fight the multiple systems of oppressions that patriarchy often intertwines itself with: racism, bigotry, homophobia, transphobia, classism, ableism, and ageism." I mean, if that's not a midlife call to action, I don't know what is.

This book is my attempt to respond to that call to action: to shine a spotlight on the radical, transformative potential of midlife. This is our chance to imagine a better world into being—and to do so in community with one another. Because it's not just about *you* doing better or *me* doing better—it's about all of us doing better together.

And so, in the pages ahead, I'll be trying to help you to make sense of all the complex and contradictory messages that our culture gives us about what it means to be a woman at midlife. I might not be able to provide you with a neat-and-tidy midlife road map, but perhaps I can help you to draw upon a few midlife navigation tools, including your inner compass. And at the same time, I'll be encouraging you to think more broadly—about other women. About imagining a better future not just for yourself, but for everyone.

CHAPTER 2

Midlife Expectations

Lola feels like she was sold a bill of goods about what midlife was going to be like. For years, the forty-four-year-old mother of three, who recently exited her second marriage, had looked forward to arriving at a stage in her life when things would somehow be easier and better. But now that she's actually arrived at midlife, she's been disappointed to discover that it isn't exactly as advertised: "You read a lot of stories in magazines about how midlife is an age of financial freedom and retirement, how easy things will be and how much we're going to love being this age, how even the sex will be better! And while there *are* some really great things about it—like, for me, caring less about what other people think—there's also a lot of hardship that goes along with it. And people don't generally talk much about that. The truth is that life isn't easier. If anything, it's more complicated. There are new levels of stress on top of the old layers of stress that you already had."

Lola isn't the only midlife woman who feels like she's been left holding an increasingly thick and messy stress sandwich, by the way. This is very much a structural issue. As feminist gerontologist Martha B. Holstein noted in a recent article for *Generations: Journal of the American Society on Aging*, the fact that women continue to take the lead on child care and elder care has far-reaching implications for their health and financial well-being, "lifetime disadvantages that no amount of individual responsibility will remedy." And as geriatric social worker and researcher Karen D. Lincoln, whose work has focused on the health and well-being of Black Americans, noted in a separate article in that same publication, the inequalities that we encounter over the course of our lives have a tendency to accumulate over time.

What adds to that stress is a set of cultural expectations about what midlife is supposed to be like—what *we're* supposed to be like by the time we arrive at this point in our lives. In this chapter, we're going to look at some of the cultural baggage the women I spoke to were carrying—and, more specifically, the expectations that made that baggage feel even heavier.

"I thought life would be so much easier by this point, but it's not."

It doesn't seem to matter exactly what your life looks like at midlife—whether you're single or in a relationship, whether you have kids or not, whether you're responsible for providing hands-on care for friends or family members or emotional support across the miles: whatever the ingredients may be in your own personal recipe for midlife, odds are there are a lot of them.

"One of the things that always gets forgotten is just how busy we are—how much responsibility is on our shoulders," says Lori, a fifty-four-year-old organizer, activist and mother of three. "There's this stereotype of the very privileged midlife woman—the Karen—who has time to have temper tantrums at the store. That caricature really ticks me off because I can only think of a handful of women I know who are even remotely like that. Most of us are totally slammed, trying to juggle everything."

Julia, a forty-seven-year-old freelance musician and mother of two, agrees. "We are the invisible glue that keeps society running.

We do all the organizing, we do all the background research and planning and we are the caregivers—of our adult children, our in-laws, our parents. We keep society running."

Basically, if you're a woman at midlife, odds are you're responsible for coordinating everyone else's life and keeping track of an incredible number of details: "Every dentist appointment; every doctor's appointment; every camp, tutoring or therapy session," explains Jodi, a fifty-year-old marketing executive and mother of teenagers. "Everything that happens behind the scenes—the scaffolding that makes my kids' lives work—is up to me. And all that work is invisible."

Invisible *and* exhausting, adds Kel, a consultant in her mid-fifties who often finds herself feeling pushed to the limit by all the competing demands on her time. She finds it desperately unfair that so much heavy lifting is left to women, noting that there simply isn't anyone else standing by, ready to step up and do that work. "If we didn't do it, who else would? Who else would work to pay half the mortgage, feed and care for everyone, clean everything? The women's movement told us we were equal but never provided the road map to achieve that equality in the home. There is still a lot of work to do on that front."

And it's not just midlife mothers who report feeling crushed by that heavy load. Alana, a forty-three-year-old government relations and policy consultant who describes herself as "a solo person, previously partnered up," feels that exact same sense of exhaustion and overwhelm: "What people get wrong about midlife is the fact that it's a slog. I think you're doing the hardest work of your life right now, whether you're a parent or not. You're worrying about elderly family members, you're potentially worrying about other people, and suddenly your health starts to become more unpredictable, on top of everything else. You can have all the confidence in the world, and you can be really proud of your achievements, but you still have to load the dishwasher, get the laundry done and figure out why your knees are aching, when sometimes you just want to sit down quietly at the end of the day and maybe not feel quite so overwhelmed."

"I had no idea there'd be so much guilt—guilt for letting myself and other people down."

Of course, where there are impossibly high expectations, there is inevitably guilt. Truckloads and truckloads of guilt. For Eileen, forty-two, the guilt is even worse than the exhaustion: "You'd think the stress would come from the fact that I'm so busy, but it's not actually that. It's the emotional turmoil, the guilt behind it all. Am I doing enough to help my son with ADHD learn strategies for living his life? Am I giving him too much attention and ignoring my other son? Have I called my mother, who lives in a nursing home, recently (in-person visits being out of the question due to the pandemic)? Do my mother's nurses understand that we don't talk as much as other families because our relationship is complicated, not because I'm an ungrateful daughter who doesn't care? Does the dog need to go out (is he suffering because he needs to pee, and I haven't taken him out enough today)? Have I done a good enough job on this work project? Oh, my husband's home now, have I spent any time on our marriage lately? My friend's house is always tidy (never mind that she has a maid and doesn't have a job), and I'm failing. We can't seriously be out of milk again; why can't I be on top of all these simple things? I'd love for someone to tell me how to let go of the guilt that I'm not doing enough or that I'm not doing it right!"

If I lived around the block from Eileen, I'd sit down with her, pour her a cup of tea and remind her that the guilt she's carrying around is terribly misplaced. It's not that she's doing it wrong; it's that she's been asked to shoulder an impossibly heavy burden—and to do so for a very long time. Just consider the number of roles and responsibilities she's juggling. When she first agreed to be interviewed for the book, she told me that she's "a wife; sister; mom of two boys (8-yr-old with ADHD, 5-yr-old neurotypical kiddo); daughter of divorced parents (a dad six hours away from me who lives alone and who I'm beginning to worry about; and a mentally ill mother who lives in a nursing home: somehow I ended up being a representative for her); volunteer nonprofit preschool board member; self-employed in a writing/editing business (part-time or full-time depends on the week)." I don't know about you, but I was exhausted by the time I finished reading her bio. Is it any wonder that she's exhausted by the day-to-day reality of living it?

And Eileen isn't alone when it comes to grappling with a crushing amount of guilt. So many of the women that I spoke with reported feeling the exact same way. No matter how much they were doing or how heavy a load they happened to be carrying, there was always this sense that they could be—and maybe *should* be—doing more.

Angela, a forty-eight-year-old author and university lecturer, has definitely felt that pressure. When she thinks back to growing up, she remembers watching her newly divorced mother scramble to re-establish her life and teaching career after stepping out of the workforce to raise kids: "She worked so incredibly hard and was part of a generation of women that did the same, setting things up so that my generation could have it all." And that's where the guilt and pressure for Angela come in: "My generation was given all these different opportunities, which made me feel like I had the obligation to take

advantage of them: the career opportunities, the parenting opportunities, the marriage opportunities. All of it."

Angela may have some very specific reasons for feeling guilty,
but it's important to recognize that just being at midlife can be
guilt-inducing in its own right. Yes, it can be a time of opportunity, but it can also be "a pressure- and guilt-filled opportunity,"
notes Alana, forty-three—a time when you can find yourself grappling with tough questions, like "Are you doing enough? Have you
achieved enough?"

Rosanna, fifty-seven, who recently retired from a corporate
career to pursue other volunteer and paid-work projects, recalls
spending entire decades of her life trying to squeeze every minute
out of every day. "I was working in a global environment so I could
work and have meetings with people at four in the morning and
then take time off during the day to take care of my kids and manage
their various appointments. I felt like I could do it all, but, as it turns
out, that's the biggest myth. You cannot do it all." A key piece of her
learning? That multi-tasking is not a real thing. "For years, I was
incredibly proud to be this multi-tasker—someone who could juggle all this stuff and feel like I had it all together. And when I look
back, that was just totally wrong." In the end, she discovered what
countless other women have figured out too: that constantly asking
your brain to toggle between different tasks isn't actually efficient
at all. It's inefficient and exhausting—and, over time, it can really
wear you down.

While multi-tasking might not be particularly effective (you're
actually making your brain work harder by constantly switching
tasks), it continues to be a much-lauded self-help strategy—the idea
being that we just have to work harder and faster so that we can
power through an impossible number of tasks all at the same time.
I don't know about you, but I can think of countless occasions when

I've tried to cook and fold laundry while carrying on a phone conversation, often to the detriment of the food I ended up scorching on the stovetop. I'm done with that. And I'm also done with other simplistic ideas about what is actually needed to achieve that magical thing called work-life balance.

Rebecca, a fifty-two-year-old social worker and single mother, is done with all that too: "The work-life balance thing is kind of a lie because it's not about organization. It's about the fact that you literally have two completely different lives and you're made to feel like you're a bad person if you're not meeting your responsibilities to everyone else in both of those lives at the same time. It's not as simple as having a schedule or doing meal prep or whatever other crazy bullshit they are telling you to do. It's more about everyone having realistic expectations about what is actually possible for a human being. And we're just not there yet."

"I thought I'd be on much more solid ground financially."

The women I interviewed for this book aren't just feeling time stressed. A lot of them are feeling financially stressed too. And even those who are on relatively solid ground financially right now can't help but worry about whether they'll be able to stay there over time.

Apparently, it's a common worry. As writer Paul Irving noted in a 2015 article for *Generations*, while older adults of previous generations worried about running out of time, the prevalent worry for today's generation of seniors is running out of money.

It practically goes without saying that the fear is a whole lot greater for women than it is for men, and for some women more than others. Audrey—who describes herself as a fifty-seven-year-old immigrant person of colour of Asian descent, a married mother of three young adults (including one set of twins) and a political party staffer—is all too familiar with that worry. Ditto for the creeping realization that, for her family at least, the much-lauded Freedom 55 lifestyle (the idea that middle adulthood is a time for reaping the rewards of all your earlier hard work by easing into a life of leisure) is proving to be more aspirational than realistic: "When I was younger, I had this idealized picture of what middle age would be like. I'd be financially secure, even comfortable, living the life that was pictured in all the advertisements—the ones that tell you, 'This is your time. You have the money to do whatever you want.' And now that I've arrived at the point in my life when all this is supposed to be happening, I'm finding that it's simply not the reality at all. Not even close.

"Sometimes I start questioning the choices I've made in my life, because other people my own age seem to be much more comfortable financially. And as for me? I don't feel comfortable at all. I feel like there's still a lot of struggle ahead. And it's not as if we've been reckless or irresponsible or anything like that. It's more a matter of life tossing us a couple of curveballs. Plus, we made some decisions—decisions that I don't regret at all, by the way—that maybe put us on a different path financially. I took eight years off of work to care for the twins when they were little, and I wouldn't trade that for anything. But by the time I went back to work, I'd lost eight pensionable years and the chance to continue to progress in my career. That translates into quite a lot of lost money. And it's yet another injustice done to women. We take time off for child-rearing, and we end up being penalized for that. It's really quite enraging if you think about it."

Joanna agrees. She's spent a lot of time crunching those numbers too—hardly surprising given the fact that she's an accountant and married mother of two in her mid-forties. Trying to combine motherhood and a career means being asked to choose between a series of less-than-great options (assuming, of course, that you even have the luxury of choice). You can continue to plow through, carrying a really heavy load, or you can decide to hit the pause button on work, thereby losing momentum on a career you might have spent more than a decade building. "They're all kind of bad choices, right?"

Add a random curveball or two, as life is apt to do, and the situation can quickly go from bad to worse. That's where Shelly finds herself these days—trying to come up with a financial plan for the years to come that takes into account the realities of her situation as a "single again" fifty-eight-year-old. "I was a child of the 1960s and a young adult in the '70s and '80s," she explains. "I thought I would get married, have a couple of kids, work for a few years, retire early and hopefully be a full-time artist by the time I was this age." What she got was "a business that failed, a marriage that failed and two children that needed way more energy than I had to give them (and I gave it to them anyway)," plus the need to exit an industry that was upended by technological change. Now she's trying to think through her options. "I don't think I'm ever going to be able to retire. I'd love to, but I don't think it's ever going to happen for me. So, right now, what I'm doing is reimagining what my sixties and seventies are going to look like. I can probably continue to do the job I'm doing right now for another ten or fifteen years, but at some point, I'm going to want to slow down, so I need to have a plan for what I'll do after that. Should I plan to do some consulting or to get a part-time job at an arts and crafts store? I think a lot of us are busy thinking through our options—recognizing that the snowbird-with-a-pension lifestyle that we saw on TV when we were kids and aspired to achieve as adults simply doesn't exist anymore."

While it may be up for debate just how much of that aspirational leisure lifestyle was actually real, it's pretty clear that the current generation of midlife adults is finding themselves on increasingly shaky ground financially—a situation that's gone from bad to worse since the Great Recession a little over a decade ago, and that certainly hasn't been helped by the far-reaching fallout from the COVID-19 pandemic. How bad has the situation gotten? Dire enough that midlife researchers like psychologist Frank J. Infurna are warning that economic pressures may contribute to "the historical worsening of mental and physical health" for the current generation of midlife adults.

Trish Hennessy shares those concerns. The director of Think Upstream, a Canadian project dedicated to policy solutions that foster a healthy society, Hennessy is also, at age fifty-five, a midlife woman herself. "So many women my age don't have a lot of income or job security. That will affect their experience as elders. And some are already being forced into a form of semi-retirement." What's needed, according to Hennessy, are policies that take into account the life trajectories of women, not just men, and that ensure that those of us who do the bulk of the care work are adequately cared for as well—that we have the financial resources we need to be able to live out the remainder of our lives in dignity.

We also need to confront the realities of the so-called gig economy—the fact that a growing number of midlife women are precariously employed, working part-time, contract or temporary jobs. These kinds of jobs can feel like the best option for women like Lola, a forty-four-year-old freelance writer with three young children, who require flexibility in order to make their lives work. But there's a downside to these kinds of arrangements, as Lola is quick to admit: "There's never an opportunity to stop working or to take time off as a freelancer. There's no paid vacation. There's no sick pay. There's no pension." The fact that she's been able to earn a really good income in a really tough profession doesn't stop her from pointing out that "the gig economy is bullshit," adding, "I don't know that I am somebody who is suited to working in an office, but I'd be a lot more sorted out financially if I had been."

Of course, having a reliable, full-time office job doesn't necessarily allow you to sidestep all that midlife worry. Alana, the forty-three-year-old government relations and policy consultant, can attest to that. "I'm very fortunate. I've worked very hard. I've had decent employment in my field for twenty-one years. And I have learned hard lessons over the last couple of years—that you can't count on your job to be there for you because at some point it won't be.

"And that precarity piece is interesting, because I find it's less tied to income and more tied to life experience. I have a decent income, but because I went through what basically amounted to a divorce ten years ago, I'm behind the eight ball financially. I don't own property—I'm a renter—so I'm not building equity in the same way as someone who owns property, and I'm increasingly being priced out of the possibility of ever being able to own a home on my own. So there's that. And then there's the fact that the future is uncertain. You may be doing well financially right now, but there is absolutely no guarantee that things will continue to play out that way. And so a lot of the work I'm doing right now at midlife is trying to figure out what I have to do over the next fifteen years so that I know I'll be okay for the following twenty."

It's a lot to think about. And forty-two-year-old Emily, for one, wishes we spent more time talking about this stuff, so that women would be less likely to blame themselves if they happen to find themselves on financially shaky ground at midlife. She's grappled with that sense of failure herself. "I feel like I failed at life a lot. Like plenty. I am a salaried, college-educated professional; I'm part of a two-income household; and I recently had to go ask my mom for money so that I could get my car fixed. I thought I would be at a different point in my life by the time I reached this age, but I'm not. I still need money from my mom. So I definitely have moments when I start second-guessing some of my earlier decisions, thinking things like, 'I should have gone to grad school.' But then I try to remind myself that this is not just about individual choices. This is not about doing the right thing or the wrong thing. There are structural issues at play—issues that impact my life and the lives of other people."

She's also the first to admit that steering clear of the quagmire of self-blame is easier said than done—and that she herself has a tendency to want to bury her head in the sand: "I have some sort of retirement fund and yet I don't ever look at it because it stresses me out too much. I'll be like, 'I know there's not enough money in there. If I look at the trajectory of that money, it's pointing straight to eating cat food when I'm ninety.' So, I don't really allow myself to think about it."

"I thought I'd finally be able to relax and coast a little career-wise."

Many of the women I interviewed for this book told me that they had expected things to get easier at work by the time they reached midlife. The expectation was that, by the time they arrived at this point in their lives, they would have proven themselves, paid their dues and earned the right to coast for a while. One high-achieving professional, who asked to remain anonymous, put it this way: "I think I thought (naively) that if I worked really hard and put in a lot of hours and effort early in my career that it would pay dividends early on and I would maybe not have to continue to pay those same dues on an ongoing basis. I'm not sure that I was necessarily thinking I'd be able to coast, but I certainly didn't expect to have to continue to grind. I still have to work really hard—harder than ever, to be honest.

I certainly didn't expect to still be putting this amount of time and effort into my career as I was heading into my fifties!"

The world of work has changed a lot in recent decades, and many of the women I interviewed are still grappling with the fallout from those changes.

For Lisa, a fifty-seven-year-old self-employed writer and editor, it has meant responding to changes in her industry: "At a time when a lot of people are gearing down, I had to gear up because the crazy industry that I decided I needed to be a part of has done a complete 180. So that's meant learning a whole bunch of new skills—and at a time when other people my age are gearing down."

For Kristine, a fifty-year-old speaker, performer and workshop facilitator, it has meant finding new ways of making a living: "When you're in your late forties, pushing fifty, good luck with that! I honestly thought that I'd snap my fingers and I'd get a new job, but that didn't happen. Employers don't want to hire middle-aged women, let alone middle-aged women of colour."

Sometimes the career challenges that women find themselves grappling with at midlife are less the result of a single dramatic curveball and more the result of a series of hard choices, the kinds of decisions that women are routinely asked to make throughout their lives and careers.

That's certainly been Kendra's experience. The fifty-three-year-old mother of three graduated with an MBA from Harvard and sky-high career aspirations: "I remember thinking that I was going to be the CEO of some cool company and that I'd be up on the stage in my suit demonstrating some exciting new product." For a while, she *did* find herself living the tech-world dream, but then a corporate merger and motherhood changed her entire career and life trajectory. She ended up taking some time off to raise her kids—a choice that was anything but validated by her former classmates:

"Imagine going to the business school reunion and feeling the conversation dead-end the moment you talked about being at home with your kids. The work that mothers do really isn't valued in our society. Raising kids who are caring people who are contributing to society—somehow, that isn't treated like it's enough." She quickly figured out that while women are told they can have it all, "you really cannot have it all and do it all at the same time, especially without support. Something's got to give. And, for a lot of us, what had to give was us. A lot of us feel disillusioned because, in having these incredibly high hopes for ourselves, we were really just setting ourselves up for failure or for exhaustion." At this point in her life, she's trying to focus less on "having an achievement I can brag about" and more on "having an intrinsic sense of value"—that inner sense that the choices she made and the life she's lived were and are enough.

"I thought midlife was supposed to be my time."

"I thought by this stage in my life, I'd be travelling, relaxing and just enjoying time with friends," says Adrienne, fifty-seven, who found herself unexpectedly single at midlife after her twenty-three-year marriage ended ten years ago. "I never expected my life to look like it does. Although I do travel, and my life is comfortable, I've come to the realization that work will continue for quite a while if I want to maintain the lifestyle I have." So much for Freedom 55.

It's not just a matter of having the funds accumulated to finance that lifestyle. You also have to have the relationship wiggle room that will allow you to take advantage of that freedom—an utter impossibility for many midlife women.

"If you're a member of the sandwich generation, like I am, you're juggling the needs of the older generation and the younger generation too," says Rosanna, fifty-seven, who recently retired from her corporate career. "I want to be able to enjoy life, and yet I've got these 'bookends' that are kind of holding me in place and, to a large degree, I can't do what I want to do because I am constrained."

"It is really a balancing act, for sure," confirms Jodi, a fifty-year-old marketing executive who is also the mother of teenagers. "You have your own goals and desire for fulfillment, but, at the same time, there are other people in your life who are counting on you."

Even if you're keenly aware of the changes you'd like to make for yourself, you still have to factor in the needs of other people. That's certainly how things played out for Jean, a fifty-three-year-old writer, academic and mother of three. "For me, the awareness that I wanted something more started peaking at a time when my parents' health was failing, and when my children were teenagers and struggling a lot more. So even as I was becoming really clear about what I wanted for myself, the demands on me were becoming much more intense and much more anxiety producing. At that point, the stakes seemed just so high: I could feel that that time was so limited, with both my parents and my children." She didn't feel she could actually start taking time for herself—pursuing her own hopes and dreams— until a few years later, after her parents had passed away and once her children weren't needing her quite so much.

Angela, a forty-three-year-old doula, yoga teacher and mother of two, looks forward to arriving at a point in her life when she has a bit more time for herself and when it might once again become possible to do something on a whim. "Things like just being able to wake up and go out for brunch and do the kinds of things that my husband and I want to do as partners. Or travelling! I do travel a lot with my children, but, even then, it still has to be something that everybody agrees on and everybody's going to enjoy. And yet there are some things that I might enjoy doing that nobody else enjoys. I look forward to someday having the freedom to just go off and maybe do some of those things, just for me."

"I thought I'd feel a lot more grown up."

Ask Alex, a psychologist who is in her mid-forties, what has surprised her the most about reaching midlife and she'll tell you it's the fact that she feels anything but grown up: "I remember back when I was younger, looking at women in their forties and their fifties, how they seemed so grown up. And now I'm that age! While on the outside I might come across as very adult and competent, inside I still feel like a kid."

Sam also admits to experiencing that same sense of disconnect between the age she *is* (forty-nine) and the age she *feels* (so much younger). "It does feel weird that my kids are old enough to leave the house, because I barely feel old enough to leave the house," she jokes. It could be because she's been immersed in the world of babies for the past two decades of her life through her role as a birth worker. These days, her job involves supporting surrogates and members of the 2SLGBTQ+ community on the journey to parenthood. "This isn't what I thought forty-nine would feel like at all. I thought it would feel a lot older."

Rather than trying to reconcile the date on her birth certificate with the way she actually feels, Leigh, a forty-seven-year-old creativity coach, has simply chosen to embrace the fact that some people continue to nurture their youthful side throughout their entire lives. "There are a lot of parts of me that haven't grown up, that still feel stuck in childhood or young adulthood," she explains. "Most often, I see this with the part of me that wants attention and recognition and to be told 'You're doing a great job.' However, being middle-aged for me means that I also have grown-up parts that have evolved to be able to see and recognize those other less-developed parts of myself. In that way, I can keep myself in check, so to speak. There's also the side of me that still loves to do cartwheels, and prank people, and laugh at crass jokes, and watch TV shows that were made for teenagers. I find that stuff harmless and amusing. It seems in defiance of what we've been told about aging and maturity, but I think it's just a well-kept secret that lots of us are still engaged with the cultural touchstones of youth. It's not just that we're trying to recapture youth or cling desperately to youth; it's that part of us still feels quite young."

Of course, there's a difference between feeling connected to your inner young person and engaging in age denialism. Rebecca, a fifty-two-year-old social worker and single mother, has watched this phenomenon play out among some of her friends: "I have a bunch of friends who are between the ages of thirty-five and fifty who don't identify as middle-aged," she explains. "And I always joke with them. I say, 'Well, how long do you think you're going to live? You're definitely in the middle of life.' They reject the term 'middle age' because they think it means you're dowdy or no longer fun. They reject that middle-aged identity for themselves." And not only do they reject that identity for themselves but they want her to reject it too. "I've been telling people I'm middle-aged since I hit thirty-five, and people will argue with me about that. I always push back when that happens because I think it's reasonable to say I'm middle-aged. I'm not at the beginning of my life. I'm having to make financial and emotional and social decisions that have to do with the middle part of my life. I'm definitely at midlife."

And even if you are willing to admit to yourself that you're venturing into midlife territory, you can still be caught off guard by the gap between midlife expectations and midlife realities. That's certainly been Andrea's experience. "I think it's a lot like motherhood," the forty-nine-year-old writer and mother of two explains. "You know about it ahead of time, but you don't *really* know what it's like until you're in it. And then when you get there yourself, it's like, 'Oh, so this is what everyone was talking about!' It feels very different from the inside out. The map is very different from the territory."

"I thought I'd have a lot more things figured out by now."

Deb, fifty-one, who is single again after being married for a five-year period in her early forties, feels a lot of pressure to have everything figured out, now that she's reached midlife. "I think that's the impression that society gives you—that, by fifty, you should have it all figured out and everything should be in place." And, by "everything," she means "a stable career and a family."

Elsa agrees. The fifty-two-year-old, who describes herself as a "career-minded Black woman," agrees. "We're given the message that we should know what we want by this point in our lives. We're told that by midlife, everything should be going great because we've lived long enough to know what we're doing. Reality is, we don't. We still don't know what we're doing."

Sadie has also picked up on the message that "you're supposed to have your shit together by midlife." And yet the front-line social service worker and activist, who is in her mid-fifties, feels like her own life is still very much a work in progress, despite a lot of ongoing effort on her part. "Just to be clear, I think I *do* have my shit together in a lot of important ways, but I don't feel like it's to the extent that society thinks I should," she explains.

Joanne, a forty-nine-year-old health-care technology entrepreneur, has a message of reassurance for other women at midlife who may be feeling pressured to magically know more than they do: "It's okay to reach this age and not have all of the answers. It's all right if your life isn't where you imagined it to be. Because you're only at the middle. There's still lots of time to love yourself and learn new things."

— CHAPTER 3 —

The Messy Middle

Suzanne remembers having big plans for herself at midlife—how she was going to celebrate this life stage. "I remember thinking, back when I was in my thirties, about how I was going to *embrace* midlife," the fifty-four-year-old Black woman, mother and grandmother recalls. "That was always my goal and my intention. I was a feminist, after all, and getting older is part of life. I had it all planned out in my head. Yes, I was going to *embrace it all.*"

And then came the midlife reality check. She discovered that midlife isn't necessarily endless bliss. Yes, it has its amazing moments, but there are a whole bunch of other kinds of moments too. "I had no idea about the physical discomforts and the emotional upheaval and how you start to become invisible," says Suzanne. "Nor did I understand that there would still be so much pressure being put on me—to be sexy, smart and able to stay on top of so many different things."

Midlife was a whole lot messier than she'd imagined.

"Midlife is magical: a time of endless possibility."

"Midlife is miserable: a time of relentless decline."

You could give yourself a bad case of cognitive whiplash trying to make sense of those two contradictory narratives about what it means to be a woman at midlife. Sure, the so-called "successful aging" narrative is a whole lot more inspiring than what gerontologists describe as "narratives of decline," but the idea that midlife is sheer magic is not without its pitfalls either.

Narratives of decline

It's not surprising that so many women head into midlife burdened by a vague sense of dread. So many of the messages that we're given by our culture encourage us to look to the future with fear. We're told, time and time again, "The best is now behind you. It's all downhill from here."

That's the biggest problem with so-called narratives of decline: they cause us to underestimate ourselves. As Margaret Morganroth Gullette notes in her book *Agewise: Fighting the New Ageism in America*, "Feeling compelled to tell a decline narrative about your one and only life is a stressor, a depressant, a psychocultural illness . . . Ageism, middle-ageism, sexism, and ableism can make those aging toward old age or chronically ill likelier to feel unwanted—unloved, sad, outcast, isolated, ashamed, helpless, and depressed, and unable to tolerate such distress."

All this is made worse by the so-called social clock, the idea that you're supposed to accomplish specific social milestones, like getting married or having children, at a particular time. Research has shown that feeling like you're not "on time" in terms of the ticking of the social clock can fuel feelings of self-doubt, incompetence and loneliness.

Elsa, fifty-two, admits to feeling seriously weighed down by what she was hearing about midlife. "I'm a Jamaican, and when I turned fifty, I was really depressed. I kept thinking about something my dad used to say to me when I was a kid: 'It's fifty up and then fifty down.' And so, when I went to my birthday party, I just kept thinking to myself, 'Oh my God, right now I'm at the pinnacle. It's all down-hill from here.'"

At the root of the problem, of course, is the fact that mainstream Western culture is obsessed with youth. And if you're treating youth as the standard, the further you move away from that standard, the less relevant you feel. It's hardly surprising that women start to feel invisible as they heed that call to take a step back and make way for the young. Culturally, you are being treated like you're invisible.

Julia, a forty-seven-year-old freelance musician and the mother of two teenagers, has picked up on that invisibility vibe too. "From the moment you turn forty, you're given the message that you need to be quiet, and you need to disappear. That's how I feel, anyway, and I'm actively working against it. I think it's harmful to society because midlife women have a lot to offer."

Emily, a forty-two-year-old professional and mother, describes it as a narrowing of possibility: "There's a narrowing there of the ways in which society allows you to be a human being, the older you get as a woman. When you're a young, single woman, there's plenty of cultural narratives out there about you. Mind you, some of them are terrible, but there are still a bunch of different ones. But the older you get, the more limited those narratives are. At this stage, it's like, 'You're a mom. That's it.' You're not given all those other ways of being. And it's very strange to me. It's just this total erasure."

"There's this sense of women at midlife losing their purpose," adds Andrea, a forty-nine-year-old writer and mother of two. "The culture tells us that we're not fertile anymore, we're not sexual any-more, we're not mothers anymore (because maybe we don't have to be mothering 24/7 at this point). There's this sense of being set adrift."

In other words, you've outlived your usefulness to the patriarchy by fulfilling your reproductive duty; now won't you please just go away? Some of the most common midlife myths seem tailor-made to support the idea that women's lives become less important—or completely irrelevant—the moment their children leave home. Take the "empty nest" myth, for example—the idea that parents are universally miserable when their offspring leave home. In fact, research shows quite the opposite: parents in general, and mothers in particular, actually report increased well-being and increased satisfaction with parenting once their kids exit the nest.

And it's not as if every midlife woman's work as a parent is anywhere close to being done. Despite what midlife myths and narratives and our culture's ticking social clock might tell us, the fact is that there's no such thing as a one-size-fits-all road map for midlife parenting (if, in fact, you end up becoming a parent at all). Some women at midlife have children who are getting ready to leave home; others have very young children who will require considerable support for many years to come. Laura, forty-seven, who is currently on leave from her job as a radio host, is definitely in the latter category: "When I turn fifty, I'll have a seven-year-old, not a twenty-one-year-old who is getting ready to leave home. I have girlfriends who are the same age as me whose kids are in their third year of university right now. And meanwhile, when I hit fifty, my son will be in grade 3."

There's also an assumption that, by midlife, the really hands-on years of parenting will be behind you and you'll be reaping the rewards of all that earlier hard work. "But sometimes things don't turn out quite that way. Sometimes there are factors that come up that derail those best-laid plans," says Sadie, fifty-three, speaking from first-hand experience. "When my kids were going through their childhood and their teen years, I think I expected that, by the time I reached this stage, there'd be some sort of payoff, for putting in all the hard work." For Sadie, parenting has required a heavy investment, both emotionally and financially. "Just in terms of the financial piece, when people start saving for their kids' future, no parent is actually thinking, 'I have to start saving because one day my child might need addiction treatment.'" And yet that's the reality for many families, including hers.

Just as frustrating as those life-limiting social scripts are the messages that tell midlife women that they no longer have anything meaningful to contribute at work—that they should just step aside and let the younger generation take over.

Lori, fifty-four, has picked up on some of those messages and she resents them. Back when she was younger, she looked forward to reaching an age when she'd finally be taken seriously. She remembered thinking, "By the time I hit midlife, I'll have earned some respect. I'll have built up the credibility that will allow me to do all the things I want to do." The organizer and activist was surprised and disappointed to discover that, when she actually arrived at midlife, her opinions simply weren't valued the way she'd hoped. "I think there's a very brief window of time when women actually have the ear of society: when they're no longer considered to be too young and before they're considered to be too old."

Ageist stereotypes about technological ineptitude only serve to make matters worse, which is why Emily, forty-two, has made a concerted effort to push back against those messages whenever she encounters them. "I was reading a book to my daughter when she was younger. It was a picture book, and it featured a mother or grandmother who couldn't figure out how to use a computer. And I felt a sudden need to stop reading the book and say to my daughter, 'Listen, I need you to know something, which is that your mother and both your grandmothers are quite capable of using a computer. I don't really know what the deal is with the woman in this book, but I just need you to know this is not typical.'"

Julia, a forty-eight-year-old small business owner and part-time university student, is convinced that these narratives of decline have gotten in the way of understanding the ability of midlife women to make meaningful contributions. "Society seems to think that midlife is when women start going downhill, physically, mentally, career-wise and in terms of participation in society. My experience has taught me quite the opposite: midlife is when women finally have an opportunity to start doing things for themselves after years and years of putting ourselves last (or at least low) on the list. There is a lot of new mental space to figure out what we want to do and how we are going to do it. Society mistakenly underestimates women at midlife."

That's one of the many reasons why Shay, forty-eight, refuses to buy into this narrative—because she refuses to sell herself short. "I don't want to be erased," she explains. "I actually like my middle-aged self better than I liked my younger self."

"Successful aging"

So narratives of decline clearly don't cut it. And the flip side of zero expectations is sky-high expectations—which is where the successful aging narrative fits in.

It's definitely a more seductive narrative than the narrative of decline, but this narrative misses the mark, too, by implying that there's a successful (and therefore also an *unsuccessful*) way to age. As cultural gerontologist Ieva Stončikaitė has pointed out, this automatically divides older people into two separate and distinct categories: winners and losers. And, honestly, who wants to fall into the category of "loser"—to be told that you're failing at midlife?

What's more, the successful aging narrative also has a tendency to treat aging as a matter of personal responsibility and individual choice (as if anyone actually "chooses" to age "unsuccessfully"). What's actually being omitted from that particular narrative is what researchers Clara W. Berridge and Marty Martinson describe as "the social, environmental, cultural, and structural contexts of aging." Erasing the impact of those broader structural factors means pretending that inequities don't exist—and it absolves governments of any responsibility for addressing those underlying issues (issues, by the way, that have a disproportionate impact on women, and women of colour in particular, as they explain). And, as if that weren't bad enough, the emphasis on personal responsibility and individual choice sets the majority of older adults up for failure by pretending that we all have the ability—and responsibility—to avoid disease, disability and functional loss, which we do not.

Once you recognize that you're being sold a rather nasty bill of goods, it becomes pretty hard to stomach the successful aging spin—the idea that something as simple as being encouraged to take charge of your own health and well-being is all that's required to age well on your own terms—a particularly prevalent and annoying message.

If we're serious about talking about aging in a way that actually acknowledges the realities of women's lives, we'll want to start by rejecting these two narrative extremes—narratives that treat midlife as little more than the beginning of the end, and narratives that pretend that there's a way to beat aging at its own game.

It's pretty clear that we need healthier alternatives to these toxic, life-limiting narratives.

So let's consider what some of those new and better midlife narratives might be.

Narratives that embrace the messy middle

Midlife isn't completely magical—nor is it completely miserable. The truth falls somewhere in the middle.

It's a point that midlife researchers like Margie E. Lachman have been trying to make for years. Sure, midlife can be a time of losses, but it's also a period of gains—and part of the challenge that we face at midlife is figuring out how to use the "assets, strengths and skills" that we've acquired along the way to compensate for or counteract some of those losses or declines.

Embracing the messy middle means acknowledging those losses and those gains in a way that allows you to find the sweet spot between feeling totally helpless and totally responsible for your own process of aging. Because, frankly, it's a much better place to be.

Grace may be someone who is relatively new to midlife (she describes herself as an academic and "a new midlife person" who recently turned forty-one), but she's already concluded that most of the traditional midlife narratives simply don't work for her. She isn't interested in totally discouraging narratives of decline, nor is she willing to buy into completely aspirational narratives that pretend that you can stop aging from happening—or that assume that preventing aging should even be a goal. "I like getting older. I am hugely relieved to be entering midlife," she explains.

Grace sees midlife as a time in our lives when we should be embracing, not fearing, just how changeable we are as humans. Instead of thinking of aging in terms of degradation or degeneration (moving further and further away from a youthful ideal), she prefers to see the process of aging as a time of "experiencing the changing self as a means to understand the world more fully." She's fascinated by the process of change and, more specifically, what it means for the lives of midlife women.

"We're so much more changeable than what we're told. I feel like it's one of the most unaddressed or uncritiqued aphorisms that's out there in popular culture, in popular science and in deep narrative. We're told that people don't fundamentally change. And yet we do. If you can recognize that of course we're constantly changing—which means that we're on these integrated physical and spiritual paths—then aging doesn't seem like a horrible thing at all."

I've spent a lot of time thinking about this conversation with Grace, as I'm sure she hoped I would. At one point, she hinted at the direction she'd like to see me go with this book: "I would love to read a book about the economics of midlife, how we understand value differently, how we value and are valued, and the tension between becoming more conservative and more radical as we are both less valued and more valued politically, economically and socially," she said. And while I didn't end up writing a book about the economics of aging (or at least I don't think I did), you'll certainly find the ideas that Grace and I talked about showing up repeatedly in this book, if only because they resonated with me on such a deep level.

This conversation inspired me, for example, to pull out my copy of Robin Wall Kimmerer's book *Braiding Sweetgrass: Indigenous Wisdom, Scientific Knowledge, and the Teachings of Plants*. Kimmerer, who is of European and Anishinaabe ancestry and an enrolled member of the Citizen Potawatomi Nation, writes about how ponds become marshes and then possibly meadows or forests, and muses about what we can learn from this as humans who are ever changing too: "Ponds grow old, and although I will, too, I like the ecological idea of aging as progressive enrichment, rather than progressive loss."

I don't know about you, but I really like that idea too—the idea of midlife as a journey of becoming. As Molly Andrews notes in her book *Narrative Imagination and Everyday Life*, "Because there is so much emphasis placed upon youth culture, there is little attention which is given to the selves we hope to grow in to, the selves we are becoming. Rarely are we asked to articulate our visions for a meaningful old age, in general, and for ourselves personally . . . Rather than restricting our thoughts on aging to strategies on how we might avoid it, we should reconceptualize it as our journey of becoming, as we grow into ourselves."

Narratives that celebrate diversity at midlife

We miss out on a lot when we try to pretend that we're all the same— or when we suggest that our journeys through midlife will be identical. I'm the kind of reader most authors have in mind when they write a book like this: a white, middle-class woman who is cisgender, married to a man, and a mother. It's pretty clear to me that we need books for and about women who don't fit that cookie-cutter image of midlife.

Women like Shay, for example. She's the forty-eight-year-old executive director of an anti-racism organization as well as a Black woman, single mother and grandmother, and she wants other people to know that middle age isn't just about white women: "I think the thing that's most frustrating to me is that the only midlife experiences that ever are validated are those of white women. There's never been a book like *Eat, Pray, Love* that's not been written about a white woman. What? Nobody thinks that women of colour have any experiences like that? It's like we don't get to have those experiences. All women—if we live long enough—go through midlife. So why is it that middle age gets centred on white women?"

It's a legitimate question, and Shay isn't the only one craving richer and more diverse midlife stories.

Emily, for one, is fed up with the broader cultural narratives that treat the nuclear family as the solution to everything. "We keep hearing that 'if you just have a family with a mom and dad and two kids, everything's going to be fine; everything's going to work out great'–and it's completely untrue!" the forty-two-year-old mother of one explains. "It's also a narrative with a really short memory: it's a made-up idea of the family that's less than a century old, but we cling to it so hard."

Lisa, a forty-four-year-old queer mother and anti-violence educator, activist and researcher, is ready to toss the nuclear family narrative out the window too. "What we learn, when we look back at history, is that humans relied on the wider community to survive. They took care of one another, lived in community and raised children together. The human race sustained itself for millennia this way because it was the most sustainable way to keep humanity alive."

And if we're getting rid of life-limiting narratives (which, of course, we are), we'll need to consider just how often midlife narratives assume that every midlife woman is part of a couple relationship and/or a mother.

Alana, forty-three, a single professional woman, knows what it's like to diverge from those mainstream narratives: "I think for single women as they age–I know myself–it always feels like people are trying to put me in a specific box to make it easier for them to understand the choices that I've made, particularly if those choices don't align with the path that they themselves have followed. I'm thinking about things like marriage, parenthood, homeownership, suburban living–all those choices that seem so traditional, depending on how you were raised. And sometimes it feels like they think I'm attacking them for making those choices.

"And then, if you happen to be a single professional woman like me, there are these conflicting sets of expectations about who you're supposed to be. Either your life is glamorous and exciting, or you're just kind of trudging along, waiting for something to change and feeling terribly disappointed in terms of where you are.

"My experience is definitely not that. I didn't necessarily plan to end up here, but I'm quite happy about where I am. So that's my experience: feeling like I'm caught between those two tropes of what it is to be a single professional woman at midlife."

Andrea, a fifty-seven-year-old geologist, has also found herself being left out of a lot of midlife narratives. In her case, she's in a long-term relationship, but she and her partner Dwayne have chosen to live apart. And she chose not to become a mother. That's meant she's been on the receiving end of a lot of judgment: "Society puts a lot of pressure on women to have kids and when you do not, you get judged."

Not every woman at midlife is a mother. And not every woman at midlife who does not have children is childless by choice. There's a difference between voluntary and involuntary childlessness—a distinction that often gets overlooked, erasing the experiences of women who had hoped to become mothers but didn't, for whatever reason.

Shauna is one of those women. "I didn't have children," the fifty-three-year-old rural resident explains. "It wasn't a choice per se because it wasn't that I didn't want to be a mom. I think I wanted to be a mom *with a partner*. But it just didn't work out in terms of timing. At that time in my life when having children might have been an option, I was either single or I wasn't with a partner I felt like I could have children with, or I simply wasn't ready. I needed to grow up a lot. I had to work on things like self-esteem, feeling worthy of a good partner, feeling worthy of having a successful professional life. So I think when my friends were busy having and bringing up children, I was busy bringing up myself."

When our midlife narratives are too limited and too limiting, we end up feeling like we're invisible or that we've failed. "If you don't see yourself, you have to work harder to convince yourself that you're all right," explains Alana, who has done a lot of thinking about this from the vantage point of a professional woman who is single at midlife.

This is why it's so important for us to share our stories—so that every woman feels seen and understood, regardless of her individual life circumstances, and so that we are exposed to a broader range of ideas about what it means to be a midlife woman. Michele, a fifty-six-year-old human resources (HR) consultant, sees this as the path forward if we want women to feel supported during this challenging time in their lives: "The more we tell our stories, the more we can push that envelope."

CHAPTER 4

Happily Stressed

"**W**hy am I not allowed to be happy?" It's a question that Beth, a fifty-year-old mother of two, has been grappling with for years, but it's become much more urgent lately. Not only has she been dealing with the garden-variety challenges of midlife, including the emotional highs and lows of raising two teenagers, but she's also been working through the emotional fallout of a corporate downsizing and the need to chart a new course for her career. It's been a lot to deal with.

As she's been busy taking stock of her current situation, she keeps bumping up against that same question. She often reflects back on a conversation she had with her father many years ago. "This was back when I was in my twenties, at an early point in my HR career, working for a really well-known company," she explains. "I told my dad that I wasn't happy with the job and that I wanted to move on. And my dad said, 'What is all this stuff about being happy?'"

For a long time, Beth thought that being happy meant doing things for other people: "'If I just do everything for everybody, they'll be happy, and then I'll be happy,' I told myself. But then I realized, 'I'm not happy.'" Because, as it turns out, endlessly trying to make other people happy is a lot of work—and it's not necessarily a ticket to your own happiness.

Fawn, a fifty-something self-employed mother of three young adults, has learned that lesson the hard way too: "It is so much work trying to please other people." It's also a strategy that is no longer working for her. "I put a fake smile on my face and try to pretend that I'm happy, but that just leaves me feeling even worse." A conversation at a funeral a couple of years back served as a wake-up call for Fawn—a reminder that she doesn't want to put her own happiness on hold indefinitely. "I started wondering if I want to spend the rest of my life focusing on the happiness of others or if it's finally time to start trying to figure out what actually makes me happy." She's still trying to find an answer to that question.

Crisis? What crisis?

Before we talk about midlife happiness, we need to tackle a midlife misconception that fuels a lot of *un*happiness. What I'm talking about, of course, is the myth of the so-called midlife crisis—the idea that crisis is an inevitable part of the midlife experience.

Given how many media articles have been written about this supposedly ubiquitous crisis (to say nothing of how many movies and novels it has inspired), you might be surprised to discover that experiencing a midlife crisis is the exception rather than the rule. As respected midlife researchers Frank J. Infurna, Denis Gerstorf and Margie E. Lachman noted in a recent article in the psychological journal *American Psychologist*, only 10 percent to 20 percent of people actually experience one.

So where exactly did we get the idea that midlife is, by definition, a time of crisis? As it turns out, from a handful of books written a few decades ago—books that really zeroed in on people who were going through times of struggle in their lives.

And then, over time, the idea of the midlife crisis kind of took on a life of its own. Ordinary people tend not only to use a much broader definition of what constitutes a crisis than the definition used by midlife researchers, but also to take liberties with the concept of midlife. As medical sociologist Elaine Wethington noted in an article written over two decades ago, when Americans are asked to describe their own midlife crises, they end up describing events that happened anytime between the ages seventeen and seventy-five—a remarkably broad definition of midlife!

But while the term "midlife crisis" may have ended up devolving into something relatively meaningless, that hasn't stopped it from continuing to cause real harm. Not only has the myth of the midlife crisis contributed to midlife's perennial image problem—the fact that most adults would rather not be middle-aged, as midlife researcher Margie E. Lachman has found—but it can also discourage midlife adults from recognizing or seeking treatment for mental health problems. After all, if you're convinced that the feelings of depression or anxiety you're struggling with are an inevitable part of life—symptoms of a supposedly unavoidable midlife crisis—you're less likely to seek treatment for those symptoms. And even if you do end up seeking treatment, you might have the misfortune of encountering a clinician who is equally invested in the midlife crisis myth and who is therefore unwilling to dig deeper to try to diagnose and treat the symptoms you're experiencing.

That's why I think we're in need of some serious cultural reframing. What if, instead of thinking "midlife crisis" we thought "midlife check-in"? What if we chose to reframe the sense of restlessness that so many people experience at midlife as something life enhancing rather than life upending? And what if we chose to treat the many turning points of midlife as opportunities for meaning making—as opportunities to reflect on our lives at this midpoint in our journeys?

"I deserve to be happy"

Lisa knows what it feels like to ask yourself tough questions. That's what her thirties were all about—engaging in the intense self-reflection that ultimately lay the groundwork for a much happier next stage of life. "By the time I reached my forties, I had started to do the work to really like myself," she explains. "I'd started to trust my instincts and to really trust myself. And I'd started to establish healthier boundaries around what felt good for me and my family, and what I simply wasn't going to put up with anymore."

At the heart of that journey were her decisions to come out as queer and to free herself from what she experienced as suffocatingly constrictive gender roles. The forty-four-year-old queer mother of two and anti-violence educator, activist and researcher explains how liberating it was to come out the other side of this experience, and how grateful she is for all the support she received along the way: "I got a lot of support and coaching from older feminists. They really validated my decision to come out of the closet at age thirty-six by helping me to understand just how common that experience is. They always talked about how every twelve years you have some sort of major disruption in your life. I don't know if that's true for other people or not, but for me it was. I had a near-death experience, and that really moved me to action. I just couldn't keep it in anymore—who I was, how I was prepared to live my life. I lost a lot of people—people I thought were my friends. And, for a while, I lost family too. But when you reach the point when you feel like it's the end of the world, when you feel like the house is on fire, there's an opportunity to resurrect like a phoenix. People really need to know that. Women really need to know that. Because it's powerful. You have the opportunity to rewrite your story, to be authentic in your body, to have boundaries that say, 'No, that's not okay for me anymore'—to say, 'This is who I am.'"

And it all starts with listening to yourself—being willing to tune in to that voice in your head that is asking tough questions and then being brave enough to seek the answers. Lisa hopes that sharing her story will encourage other women to do just that: "I hope that women out there are able to listen to that gut feeling that says there's something not right here, that I deserve to be happy, at least some of the time. I deserve to be able to feel joy. And I am worthy."

Feeling all the feelings

So what does it take to journey to that happier place? For some women, it starts with allowing themselves to acknowledge, perhaps for the first time ever, the depth and range of emotions they are feeling.

For Kendra, fifty-three, a married mother of three with an MBA from Harvard, that has meant allowing herself to feel all the feelings as opposed to just a narrow range of emotions that she grew up believing were acceptable. "The more in tune I've become with my own body, the more I've realized there were a lot of feelings in there that I wasn't acknowledging. So that's been kind of mind-blowing," she explains.

Sadie, a front-line social service worker and activist in her mid-fifties, has been going through a similar process, learning to accept the wide range of emotions triggered by her daughter's mental health and addiction struggles. "At midlife, I have found a way to hold the grief and pain and also be able to lean in close for the love and laughter. At earlier stages of my life, I would not have thought these feelings could co-exist. I would not have thought it would be possible—or desirable—for me to be happy while one of my children continues to struggle. I would not have thought I could have this much compassion for a person whose actions continue to break my heart."

As a result of a lot of hard work, to say nothing of therapy, she's acquired a set of emotional management skills that she can draw upon to weather life's many storms. "I found individual therapy really, really helpful," she explains. "I've found some very specific resources that have been really key, and the main one is the concept of radical acceptance, a key concept in dialectical behavioural therapy. That has been huge for me—to see that I can accept the reality of the situation I'm in without necessarily being okay with it. I can still feel hurt and frustrated and all sorts of other things about it, but I suffer less when I allow myself to acknowledge the reality of what I'm dealing with and to name it."

She's also learned how to analyze her own thinking patterns—and, more specifically, to recognize when her thinking is becoming more rigid and less nuanced, something that typically happens when she finds herself in crisis mode: "Through therapy, I've learned to spot when this is happening, and I've learned how to push back against that tendency. This has taught me that it's possible to exercise some control over how I feel about what's happening in my life. Practices such as radical acceptance (and yes, it is a practice that takes work) help to calm my nervous system, and that in turn allows me to think more flexibly, so that I don't get locked into specific ways of reacting; I'm able to maintain a more nuanced view of the situation, and I have more space for compassion and genuine connection. This helps me to recognize that, even when I feel stuck, I still have choices about how to react, and I have more internal resources than I might have otherwise expected. Radical acceptance helps me to see that, in fact, even with this wild and crazy situation, I still have some control."

The truth about midlife happiness
(and unhappiness)

The midlife crisis isn't the only myth to oversimplify our complex relationship with happiness (or unhappiness) at midlife, to make it difficult for us to fully acknowledge the range of emotions that we might be experiencing. The U-curve of happiness has also contributed to the confusion. What I'm talking about here is a theory put forth by British-American labour economist and researcher David Blanchflower. Blanchflower has tried to make the case that happiness levels decline during a person's twenties, thirties and forties; bottom out between the ages of forty-seven and forty-nine; and then rise again as that person heads into later life.

It's a compelling theory—one that the mainstream media totally loves, by the way—but it doesn't really stand up under scrutiny. And Blanchflower has certainly been on the receiving end of a lot of criticism. Critics have argued that the U-curve may be more of a baby boomer phenomenon than a more generalizable midlife phenomenon that applies to people of different generations. They've pointed out that the theory tends to overemphasize a single ingredient in the recipe for happiness in a way that distorts the findings: while life satisfaction reaches a low point at midlife, other psychological constructs, like the amount of positive emotion, actually show a steady rise from youth through old age. Critics have also suggested that the U-shaped pattern may be more about the dip in marital satisfaction that is known to happen during the really hands-on years of child-rearing than anything else. But the most pointed critique is simply that the study design itself is flawed. It's generally more valuable to track the life experiences of the same group of people over time than to consider the experiences of an ever-changing pool of people (by comparing, for example, people who were at midlife thirty years ago with people who are at midlife today).

I'll save you the trouble of poring through dozens of psychological studies (although they do make for pretty great reading, if you're the kind of person who appreciates a good old-fashioned academic brawl): all you really need to know about the controversy is that Blanchflower's theory has been largely debunked. As Jeffrey Jensen Arnett put it in a 2018 article, there's little support for the claim that midlife is "a slough of despond to be glumly endured," and that it's perhaps both misguided and simplistic to try to make the case that midlife is either positive or negative overall. Because is anything about midlife that neat and tidy? At this point in the book, you know that the answer is a firm no.

Attempting to reduce something as complex as human emotion to a predictable pattern that you could expect to observe in some "typical" (and mythical) midlife person does seem to be a pretty meaningless exercise, especially given that the data appears to hide more than it reveals. As you might expect, there are significant demographic disparities when it comes to the midlife experience of happiness, as Phyllis Moen points out in her book *Encore Adulthood: Boomers on the Edge of Risk, Renewal, and Purpose*. "White men in their fifties, sixties, and early seventies have the greatest odds of being very happy, followed by white women, then black men, and finally black women," she notes.

What makes it even more complicated is the fact that contemporary ideas of happiness are so anchored in ideas of personal responsibility and individual achievement. And if your yardstick for happiness involves constantly scrambling to stay one step ahead of everyone else, it's pretty hard to find happiness at *any* life stage, let alone midlife.

My advice? Lose that yardstick and replace it with a better one—one that emphasizes meaning making and finding a sense of purpose, a recognition that true happiness emerges from "the depth of our moral concerns and commitments" and our willingness to intertwine our emotional lives with others', as Simon Fraser University professor Jeff Sugarman put it in an article in the *Journal of Theoretical and Philosophical Psychology*.

Now that's a definition of happiness that can lead to the real deal. And it's what we're going to spend a significant portion of the remaining chapters of this book talking about—the joy of journeying through midlife in the company of others.

Happily stressed

Of course, none of this discussion of happiness is an attempt to minimize the extent of the struggle for many midlife adults. Midlife can be a crunch time on so many fronts. As Margie E. Lachman has noted, midlife is a time in your life when there's too much to do and not enough time.

And it's not as if this situation is likely to improve anytime soon. If anything, things are getting worse. Just think about the cultural moment that we're living through—the climate crisis, the pandemic, the widespread social and political upheaval. Clearly, all of that is having an impact, too, at some broader cultural level. That's definitely Jean's take on the matter. "I see people around me who I think are probably going through a midlife crisis. And sometimes I look at our country and I think *it* might be going through a midlife crisis. It doesn't know who it is. It doesn't know what it wants. It's freaking out," says the fifty-three-year-old writer, academic and mother.

The research makes it pretty clear that "crisis" isn't the right word to describe this midlife state of affairs.

And that maybe "happiness" isn't the right word either.

We need something that's both messier and a lot more honest, something that hints at all that messiness.

Maybe we need to pick up on a phrase that developmental psychologist Jeffrey Jensen Arnett coined a couple of years ago. That term is "happily stressed."

As he explained in a 2018 article, most midlife adults aren't completely happy, nor are they completely unhappy. We're neither in a perpetual state of crisis nor are we perpetually stress-free. It may be that what most of us end up experiencing in our lives can best be conceived of as more of a hybrid experience: one part happy and one part stressed. *Happily stressed*, in other words.

CHAPTER 5

The View from Midlife

Tricia found herself going through a period of intense intro-spection around the time of her fiftieth birthday—an event she describes as a landmark life event. "It's like when you're looking for a way to get somewhere, you're always looking for those landmarks, like, 'Turn left at the old schoolhouse.' So, I guess I kind of felt like fifty was my old schoolhouse," she explains.

Making plans for her birthday got her thinking about "who I was, how I got here and what I've achieved" and remembering "what it felt like to be that little kid who just wanted to help people."

That journey down memory lane helped her to recognize how little she valued that trait—that hard-wired essence of kindness—in herself when she was younger: "I remember when I graduated from high school, they were giving out all these awards. There are academic awards and sports awards and then there was the award I ended up sharing with another student: the congeniality award. And, at the time, I remember thinking, 'This is terrible. What if all I ever end up being is a nice person?' Like that was a bad thing!"

But now, with a couple of additional decades of living under her belt, she's come to appreciate that quality in herself—the way kindness has ended up being a thread that holds together her entire life story. "I've never been someone to just sit back. I've always been someone who wanted to connect with and care for people. And now that I'm fifty and doing some of that reflection, I'm able to see how, in many ways, I've continued to be that same person. I can see how, all the way along, I was who I truly was."

A midlife identity quest

Midlife is a time of self-reflection, a time in your life when you're likely to find yourself thinking about who you've been, who you are and who you are becoming. In the words of midlife scholar Sharon Wray, it's a time when "past, present and future intersect."

At midlife, we've reached a point in our lives where our brains have accumulated a lot of knowledge and experience. They've also become really good at making connections and spotting patterns in a way that helps our lives to make sense, both looking backward and looking forward. Perhaps that helps to explain the busyness of our midlife brains—what Susan describes as "that feeling that your brain is out of control." The forty-five-year-old writer, coach and mother has spent a lot of time wondering about the energy of the midlife brain—her brain as well as the brains of other women she knows. "I'm honestly curious to see if there's anything neurological happening, because it feels like a storm, and it seems to be happening to almost everybody I know. There must be something going on. It feels so physical."

If that sense of restlessness and curiosity sounds familiar, it's because you've been here before. You're basically revisiting the identity quest of adolescence. In her book *Composing a Further Life: The Age of Active Wisdom*, Mary Catherine Bateson highlights the similarities between these two introspectively demanding life stages: "The challenges that lie ahead at fifty and sixty are those that we encountered at sixteen and twenty-five: discovering who, finally, I am, who and what I am able to commit to, how to sustain that commitment, and how to invest my energy and my caring."

The good news is that, as women, we've had lots of practice when it comes to reinventing ourselves. Andrea, a forty-nine-year-old writer and mother of two, explains: "I think that women—and especially women who are mothers—go through these kinds of identity shifts in a way that men just don't. We have to shift our identities when we become mothers. When we become mothers of teenagers, we have to shift our identities again. And then again when we become mothers whose children don't live at home anymore, or even children who aren't alive anymore. We have to shift our identities. We're shape-shifters in that way."

Lara, forty-seven, who describes herself as "a military wife, mother to an atypical teen, a teacher, Indigenous—Secwépemc-Métis—and a survivor of both PTSD [post-traumatic stress disorder] and the Sixties Scoop," can relate to the whole concept of shape-shifting. That's been the theme of the past few decades of her life: "Life took some unexpected turns and I had to recalibrate myself a number of times. Losing my childhood family required me to do a reset of who and what is important to me. Not being accepted by my biological family forced me into another reset. I had to redefine who I was when my pelvis broke, and I was no longer the active, agile, self-sufficient person I saw myself as. Realizing that my child had special needs further changed my reality and who I am. Every speed bump or hurdle has encouraged me to pause and reflect."

The challenge, of course, is finding the time and space needed to take that pause—no easy task during what can be an exceptionally busy life stage and when you're living in a culture that prioritizes *doing* at the expense of *being*. Sometimes you have to look for opportunities—even just small moments—to create that pause for yourself, taking into account the realities of your life and what is reasonable or even possible for you right now.

For Christine Luckasavitch, an Indigenous author, scholar and cultural consultant, that means recognizing the value of that pause and knowing herself well enough to recognize what will be most restorative. "For me, it's going outside for a ten-minute walk: just being quiet and being in nature. It could be just stopping to listen to the sound of the lake, or to the sounds of the chickadees that are so busy right now." Not only is this time calming and restorative, but it also helps to forge a healing relationship with nature—with all your non-human relations. "Your relations are there to support you, to uphold you, when you need that pause and when you need that nourishment the most," she explains.

If Christine is passionate about this, it's for good reason. She feels a deep connection to the land—and, more specifically, the land that has been part of her family's story since time immemorial. She's an Omàmìwininì Madaoueskarini Anishinaabekwe (a woman of the Madawaska River Algonquin people) and of mixed settler heritage. She told me about a time in her life—a really difficult time, when she had just exited a bad long-term relationship—when walking the same path on a daily basis over a period of months ended up being both an exercise in noticing and a ritual of comfort. She explains: "What I did was move to a place that had been in my family for a very long time. And I ended up walking pretty much the same path every single day. I started in mid-spring, and I was able to keep doing it until the end of August. That gave me an opportunity to really observe the changes that were happening day to day in just that small, small span of the land, to see how plants go from being small to producing fruit to being eaten or preparing for the next season or the next phase of that plant's life. What you begin to see is that there are all these cycles happening in nature all the time. You just have to pause and notice them. And that can be really comforting, even healing."

Christine's experience really speaks to that need for pause: how important it is to look for tiny opportunities in your day-to-day life to both reconnect with and nourish yourself. It's all about building a relationship with yourself that's rooted in self-compassion and self-understanding, knowing yourself well enough to recognize what you need and loving yourself enough to try to meet that need.

And it's also about opening your eyes to the bigger picture: understanding who you are, and how you fit into the world, as you pause to take in the view from midlife.

Reconnecting with your younger self

For Joanna, midlife has been a time for reconnecting with her younger self. "It's sort of like a bit of a zooming out, looking back in time and being curious about who I was then, because I'm still that same person at my core," the forty-six-year-old accountant and mother of two explains.

She's particularly drawn to a specific moment in her life, when she was invited to be part of a month-long international peace and justice tour at the age of thirteen. "I was the youngest person on that tour," she explains. "They had brought together about seventy young people between the ages of thirteen and twenty-six from all around the world. It ended up being a transformative experience—one that I reflect on a lot. Where did that young, idealistic girl think she would be thirty years later? What would she think of the person I've become? Would I measure up? Would she be proud of me? Would she feel disappointed in me for 'settling'?"

While a lot of women like to imagine themselves having that kind of conversation with their younger selves, Emily's been able to take things one step further. She's had the opportunity to get reacquainted with her younger self via her childhood diary. From the vantage point of age forty-two, she has been shocked to discover just how much of a disconnect there is between the way she has come to remember her childhood and the thoughts and experiences she recorded in her diary at the time. "It's fascinating to see how the things I've chosen to remember about myself or know about myself compare to what I actually wrote down back then. I think of my childhood as being a very happy time. I have really positive memories of growing up. I had a good relationship with my parents. I had a happy childhood. But then I go back and read my diary and I keep coming across all these things that I was really angry about. It's really interesting to me to see how much I have set aside those angers and frustrations over the years, so that I could arrive at a place where I could say, 'I was a happy kid,' when, in truth, it's more like, 'No, you were seriously a really angry kid: a kid who was actually angry about a lot of things.' That's fascinating to me."

Like Emily, Susan has been engaging in some midlife time travel. She's been trying to solve a few mysteries—to make sense of the life-upending series of events that had her family packing up and moving on a regular basis. "In the first twenty-two years of my life, I lived in twelve different towns on three different continents: [in] Canada, England and South Africa," the forty-five-year-old writer, coach and mother explains, joking, "My parents really squeezed all the juice out of the Commonwealth!" It wasn't until she was an adult herself that she started questioning the narrative she'd grown up with. "My parents basically framed moving to Canada as an adventure. I thought we were just kind of a fun family who didn't like to stick around for too long. But, in a lot of ways, it was fleeing. My father was running away from mistakes he had made at the time, and he was always trying to find a place where he would feel comfortable with himself. Unfortunately, it didn't work." It wasn't until after both of her parents had died and Susan was sorting through her mother's things that she was finally able to put together the pieces of her family's story in a way that actually made sense. Suddenly, she was able to understand things in a way that simply hadn't been possible when she was younger.

Lara, forty-seven, can relate to that midlife search for answers. In her case, the search has focused on issues of identity related to her adoption by a non-Indigenous family. She explains: "I got a bit of a late start in terms of figuring out who I am. I didn't learn a lot of my family history until I was in my thirties, and what I did learn at that point (that I was part of the Sixties Scoop) changed a lot about my understanding of who I am as a person. We live our own stories, but those stories are flavoured by those around us and often structured by who or what came before us. And so I find myself in the unusual position of figuring all this out as an adult. Not just learning *who* I am as a person, but learning my family history, my story."

Lisa's midlife has also been centred on the experience of solving a long-standing family mystery related to her adoption. While she'd grown up knowing that she was adopted, it wasn't until 2018, when the province where she was born changed its privacy laws regarding adoption records, that Lisa (who was then in her mid-fifties) was able to start figuring things out: "Suddenly, I had names." With help from members of a Facebook group, she was able to track down copies of her parents' obituaries, which, in turn, provided her with the names of other members of her birth family. She ended up making contact with one of her half-sisters and connecting with other members of her extended family, a process that yielded some welcome health information and allowed her to forge relationships with some of the members of her birth family. As she likes to put it, "I've added a couple of twigs to the family tree."

Jude, a post-secondary administrator in their early forties who describes themselves as non-binary agender, has been engaged in a similar process of filling in some gaps in their family tree. "I grew up with ghosts," Jude explains. "I had three older half-sisters that were adults or nearly adults when I was born. They were not around when I was growing up, and there was the unspoken rule that we were not to talk about them, even though their childhood photos were on display. My dad had five kids over twenty-six years and he didn't get any better at parenting over the years." A series of events allowed Jude to connect with some of those siblings in recent years. They're still trying to figure things out as a family. "How does one create a relationship with siblings, from scratch, after thirty-five years of estrangement? I don't know. It's been a few years and I still don't know." The situation elicits a lot of feelings of sadness and regret for Jude. "I wish so much that these people had always been part of my life, especially as I struggled as a single parent and could have used the support of family, of sisters who were also single parents."

Making peace with the past

While childhood and adolescence may feel long ago and far away for many, for some they are still full of unanswered questions or unresolved issues. As Sadie puts it, "I'm in my mid-fifties and I'm still really impacted by dynamics from my childhood."

Beth feels that impact too. Her dad had a high profile in the community and Beth grew up understanding that she was expected to live by a very rigid set of rules: "I couldn't wear jeans, I couldn't wear track pants and I couldn't wear makeup because I was this person's kid. I remember feeling like I wasn't actually allowed to be me: I was someone's kid and I had to behave in a certain way." While she's finally reached a point in her life where she's emotionally ready to acknowledge the impact of those family rules, she's also quick to stress the fact that she doesn't blame her parents for the far-reaching psychological fallout of her childhood. "I accept that my parents are themselves children of parents"–other imperfect parents. "My parents didn't do anything intentionally. They learned what they learned, and they passed it on to me."

Kendra, fifty-three, has also been thinking about how much of her life has been devoted to doing things to impress other people. It's a pattern that was established back in childhood and grew from a desire to follow in the footsteps of a father she both admired and adored: "My dad is an economics professor who specializes in finance, so our dinner-table conversations were always about economics and entre-preneurship." When Kendra headed off to college, she chose to major in economics and then to head off to business school, "all because of his encouragement." She also notes that the career decisions she made were also very much a product of the times. The 1980s was a decade when achievement and success were glorified, and so choosing to go to Harvard to get an MBA left her feeling like she was "checking all the boxes" in terms of both achievement and success. "What I have real-ized as I've gotten older is that I was doing so much to please him and to check those boxes that I kind of lost track of what I wanted. I hadn't realized until very recently how many parts of myself I ignored while I was pursuing those other things–making those other choices that I knew would impress other people. And so it has taken probably the past ten years of my life for me to really become myself. I had no idea that, at midlife, I would still be becoming myself."

For Shay, a forty-eight-year-old Black woman, midlife has been an awakening–a time when she's become really comfortable speaking her truth. "I don't need people to like me," she explains. "I know I'm not everybody's cup of tea and that's fine." She wishes that more women—and white women in particular—could find a way to break free of the need to be liked by other people. She sees it as one of the more toxic elements of white culture—one that discourages independent thinking and prevents women from growing into the fullest versions of themselves: "I think that people pleasing is very much part of the way that white women are raised, and even at mid-life, they say things like, 'I have to try.' And to that I say, 'No, actually, you don't. You don't have to try to make people like you.'"

Emily, forty-two, has equally strong feelings about some of the cultural scripts that were dumped in her lap back when she was a younger woman. She remembers struggling with the conflicting messages she was being given about white womanhood, and femininity in particular. "I grew up with a mom who did not embrace the feminine," she explains. "And I think I absorbed some ideas about femininity, as a result of growing up in that environment, a situation which proved to be really challenging as I grew into being a woman. I grew up hearing that if you performed femininity in a particular way—if you were conventionally attractive, cared about your appearance, and if you wore makeup and did your hair—it was because you weren't very smart."

Emily remembers experiencing a lot of "cognitive dissonance" around these messages: "I was a very bright kid who did well in school and loved to read—but I was also interested in fashion when I was growing up." She couldn't figure out why she was being asked to choose one script or the other—why she was only allowed to be pretty *or* smart—why she wasn't allowed to imagine herself being both these things. "And I still feel like I'm banging my head up against that idea. I feel like I see news headlines every couple of weeks that reinforce that binary. I'm raising a daughter, and it's so hard for me to find that middle path, for her or for me. What does that even look like?"

She's been equally eager to ditch another toxic piece of cultural baggage that she encountered during her growing-up years: the obligation to treat yourself as a perpetual self-improvement project. "I remember getting that message so many times as a kid—that you have to fix yourself and become a certain thing—and then (but only then!) you would be worthy. And, once again, these ideas of worthiness were packaged in one of those narrow roles. There were only a few ways to be a woman and you had to pick one and then do the work to get yourself there. And the underlying message was always 'Whatever you are right now, it's not enough. You're not good enough or even okay.'"

This kind of deep introspection and soul searching—a willingness to question everything about your culture, your past experiences and yourself—demands a tremendous amount of self-knowledge and self-trust. Perhaps that's why it tends to happen at midlife: we finally know ourselves and trust ourselves enough to be ready to do this work. Finally, we feel brave enough to acknowledge where we've been, who we are and where we're headed next—to chart a course to a happier, healthier place.

Self-compassionate remembering

Few of us manage to arrive at midlife without accumulating at least a few regrets. And so, for some of us, midlife is a time for making peace with the past and finding a way to come to terms with some of the difficult decisions we might have had to make along the way.

For Rebecca, a fifty-two-year-old mother of two, that's meant grappling with some post-divorce regrets: "My regret is that maybe for the sake of my kids and for the sake of the stability of the household, I should have stuck it out in the marriage. I regret some of the stuff that my kids went through having to do with our divorce—feeling insecure. I regret that that part of their childhood was painful—and that we were poor. If Steve and I had stayed together, we probably could have enjoyed things like vacations. And I probably could have still lived my life within the confines or the disappointments of that marriage."

Leaving a marriage is a high-stakes decision—and one with far-reaching consequences. Making peace with a decision like this one often involves treating yourself with compassion, recognizing that you made the best possible decision you could with the information and options you had at the time. Because, if you think about it, what more can you ask of yourself? As Nancy Mandell, Susannah Wilson and Ann Duffy note in their book *Connection, Compromise, and Control: Canadian Women Discuss Midlife*, "Women make the best possible choices they can under difficult circumstances; these so-called 'choices' often do not appear immediately significant but in fact set in place a series of other consequences that resonate throughout their lives in often unexpected and sometimes uncontrollable ways. Midlife is all about reflecting on this chain of events, of trying to make sense of how the pieces fit together, and then coming to a place of acceptance."

Sometimes that means making a conscious decision to tell a particular story in a more self-compassionate way. It's one of the great things about being human: we're constantly editing the stories we tell ourselves about our lives. And as our stories change, we change too.

This, of course, is the magic of life review. It can be a path to self-forgiveness and even healing. As Sara Ruddick noted, in a contribution to Margaret Urban Walker's book *Mother Time: Women, Aging, and Ethics*, "There is a sense in which the past is not unalterable but can be remade through focused remembering. Notoriously, memories are deeply felt, but their meaning is neither static nor self-evident . . . Without denying facts or pain, a person may actually remember more compassionately, with a sharper sense of context and complexity."

This process of compassionate remembering can result in a growing sense of self-knowledge, and an appreciation for the hard-earned wisdom you've acquired along the way.

In her book *Awakening at Midlife: A Guide to Reviving Your Spirit, Recreating Your Life, and Returning to Your Truest Self*, Kathleen A. Brehony offers this helpful analogy: "[Nineteenth-century philosopher Arthur] Schopenhauer compared life to a piece of embroidery: during the first half we look at the right side, while during the second half we see the wrong side—which, he points out, is not as beautiful but is more instructive, since we can see the way in which the threads have been worked together."

Sure, there's been a lot of messiness, but there's also been a lot of beauty.

CHAPTER 6

Self-Acceptance: The Midlife Edition

There's a long list of things to love about midlife, but at the top of the list for a lot of women is a growing sense of self-acceptance. There's something tremendously liberating about finally understanding and embracing who you truly are. This is something Junia has spent the past few years discovering. She isn't just new to the experience of being at midlife; she's also new to the experience of living as a woman. A month after coming out as a transgender woman, the forty-two-year-old was fired from her job as a pastor at a suburban Baptist church. But while her midlife journey of self-acceptance has been particularly far-reaching and high-stakes, Junia is finding a lot of common ground with other midlife women.

"I guess one of the things I've picked up from talking to middle-aged women is that there's often this sense that you're coming out of a period of your life where you've lived according to other people's expectations," she explains. "And then, at some point, you decide that you're tired of living that way. And I think that's where the experience of a transgender woman transitioning in life is so similar to that of every woman. There are so many things that we're told we have to be, so many things that we're told we can't be, and sometimes it takes us a while to break those chains. And those first steps of freedom can be really terrifying.

"But, to put a theological face on it, I think that's what we were created to do and who we were created to be. So, whether that means you've spent the first forty years of your life living in the wrong gender or married to the wrong person or in the wrong career, it's okay to get to this point in your life and say, 'You know what? I'm done with that. I'm just going to be myself.' And that's what I'm trying to do, day by day."

Arriving at a place of self-acceptance

So how do you find your way to this magical place of self-acceptance? (Because getting there really does feel magical, even if you only manage to visit occasionally at first.) For a lot of women, it means making a decision to recognize and honour who you truly are.

"You start to know yourself better," explains Alana, forty-two. "You have a better sense of what you are—and aren't—willing to tolerate. You have a bit more confidence in the decisions you're making for yourself. And, if you're really lucky, maybe you get to live your truth a little more."

For Alex, who is in her mid-forties, living that truth means noticing how much her priorities have shifted in recent years. She's still juggling a lot of responsibilities—a psychology practice, teaching responsibilities at a university and the day-to-day demands of single parenthood—but now her emphasis is less on achievement and more on contribution: "I'm not so interested in impressing anybody anymore. I don't have time for that. I don't want any gold stars. I just want to do my work and bring my tiny little gift to the world."

For other women, it's also about rejecting a lot of external expectations that simply aren't working for them anymore—assuming, of course, that they ever worked for them in the first place.

Alex (in this case, a different Alex) recalls just how crushing those expectations felt for her for so many years. In fact, the forty-five-year-old entrepreneur, who found herself "suddenly divorced" five years ago, can still recite those sky-high expectations in the playbook for suburban womanhood from memory: "You'd better have a tidy house. Your kids had better know how to read by the time they start school. You'd better have a great marriage (which means you'd better be sleeping together on a regular basis, even after ten years of marriage). And you'd better be finding a way to spend time with your friends." It felt like a lot ("I don't know how people get through it sanely," she says), but she didn't feel like she had any choice but to keep trying to live by those rules. "And, sure, people would try to tell me that it's okay to let go of things or to settle for good enough, but, honestly, that was bullshit, because whenever I went to their houses, everything was perfect. There was no way I could be the messy one." Then, one day, everything changed, including her. "Maybe it was the end of my marriage that finally allowed me to have the freedom to let that stuff go," she says. Instead of worrying about playing by that old set of rules, she's writing a new post-divorce playbook for herself—one that spells out how she chooses to live her life: "I get to make these kinds of decisions for myself, and, honestly, it feels so free."

It can be tremendously liberating to suddenly discover that you care less about what other people think—that you are able to let go of so many external pressures and expectations. Journalist and broadcaster Nana aba, forty-three, is looking forward to experiencing some of that midlife liberation too. "The idea of coming into a stage where I really don't care what other people think sounds so tantalizing," she says. And while she might not be quite there yet, she's definitely on her way. In fact, she's been on her way for a while. "Once I had children, I started to understand the no-nonsense attitude of some women. I started to realize that what it often comes down to is time: you literally do not have time to care about a lot of things."

For Lola, forty-four, arriving at that place of self-acceptance has meant circling back to an earlier time in her life and reconnecting with her younger, feistier self: "I think fundamentally I'm very much the same person, but I feel like I have had to shake off the conditioning that was put on me by my parents, by society, by men, by all the roles I was expected to take on." And yet, at her core, there has always been this rebel spirit whose heart burned with a fierce sense of justice. "When I was a kid, my mother used to [joke about how] I was always out there demonstrating for some socialist kind of cause, fighting the good fight. I've always been that person," she recalls. And that's the part of herself that she's always really liked—and that she's proud to see reawakening again. "These days, I like myself a lot. In many ways, it feels like I'm coming back to maybe a purer version of who I was."

Like Lola, Jennifer, a forty-eight-year-old divorce coach, is no longer willing to hide who she is: "I've learned to embrace who I am. For so long, I tried to tamp down who I was to accommodate the wishes of others. I no longer hide the masculine energy that makes me good in business, just so the men around me feel okay. I embrace my feminine energy (I adore fashion and design) without feeling that doing so makes me seem less serious. I'm not everybody's cup of tea and it's taken me almost fifty years to realize that's quite okay."

Tapping into all that hard-won self-knowledge

Often the first step toward self-acceptance is self-knowledge—and once you know yourself better, you can learn to embrace your own glorious imperfection (as opposed to running from it), opening the door to so much possibility. Instead of being afraid of being wrong, you can become more comfortable with making mistakes or not knowing.

That's what Suzanne, fifty-four, has discovered in recent years. Instead of putting pressure on herself to become someone she isn't, she's chosen to both capitalize on her strengths and compensate for her weaknesses. The birth worker, single parent and grandmother explains: "When I was younger, I felt that certain things should come naturally to me. I should be naturally organized. I should be naturally tidy. I should naturally be motivated to do the things that I need to do, like exercising. But with age has come a huge amount of self-acceptance. I recognize that I'm never going to be that neat, organized and highly motivated person naturally. I need to have systems in place to ensure that I get things done. I need planners and agendas. I need lists. I need routines and schedules. And they need to be fairly strict because if I don't keep myself in line, then everything falls apart. I'm the kind of person who needs preauthorized payments for her rent and her car payments. Otherwise, none of my bills would get paid. And I need to have a reason to go for a walk. That's one of the reasons I ended up getting a puppy!"

"When I was twenty, I thought I knew everything," says Shelley, a forty-nine-year-old writer, communications instructor and bookstore employee. "I honestly thought I knew it all. But now that I'm approaching fifty, I'm becoming really comfortable with the idea that there's a lot I don't know and a lot I don't understand. And I'm good with that."

For Lisa, a forty-seven-year-old who describes herself as "gender queer, pansexual, a mom of two, an activist and an activist scholar," being at midlife means learning to appreciate nuance and contradiction: "I think that, at midlife, we start to recognize that things are rarely black and white. Every issue, every situation, is incredibly complex and nuanced." And with that realization comes freedom: the freedom to not have to be right all the time. "Sometimes you'll be right and sometimes other people will be right—and that's okay." That willingness to be wrong unlocks a world of possibility for yourself and other people, an invitation to learn and grow together.

Seeing and celebrating your many strengths

The view from midlife can be pretty spectacular: it's a chance to reflect on how far you've travelled, how much you've lived through and how much you've learned.

Often it's the hardest legs of the journey that end up teaching you the most about yourself. Here's how Claire, a forty-year-old Black woman who is also a mother of two and the founder of a non-profit organization, puts it: "Success and thriving, in the end, is not from the easy moments. It's in overcoming those mountains that seem so insurmountable. And even if you don't actually manage to make it all the way over those mountains, you can still look down and say, 'Look how far I've come.'"

Like many women at midlife, Shymol—an engineer in her fifties—has climbed a lot of mountains. It's a journey that started with her decision to emigrate to Canada from India twenty years ago—a decision that felt both urgent and necessary at the time. "If you are a woman growing up in India, your life is everybody's business right from childhood until you die. What you wear, what you do, what you think or don't think: all of this has to be permitted by the men of the family and society." While she was lucky enough to grow up in a progressive family that granted her a fair bit of freedom, she wanted so much more for herself. "I didn't have it in me to constantly defy these norms, so I chose to migrate to a free country like Canada. And it was one of the best decisions of my life." Looking back, she is in awe of her younger self, being willing to take that on. "There were many challenges: language barriers in terms of accents, cultural issues, finding a job before the money ran out. Uprooting to come to a new country alone is a hard decision." She is also proud of herself for finding the courage to leave an abusive marriage, and to rebuild her life as a single parent. Midlife, for her, is proving to be a time of celebration: "At this stage of life, there is a sense of content, sense of peace, sense of courage to enjoy life's little moments. It is hard to put it into words."

Like Shymol, Shauna, fifty-three, is proud of the person she has become as a result of coming through earlier times of struggle. "I have been without work for long stretches of time. I actually had to be on social assistance for a while. But I'm also really resilient. I just keep going." She doesn't just see that as a matter of personal strength, by the way: she's quick to acknowledge that she benefited from a combination of luck and privilege, that her story might otherwise have turned out a very different way. She's also moved beyond the point of blaming other people for the hard things she experienced, choosing instead to feel grateful for the learning and growth that happened as a result of living through those earlier experiences. She explains: "When I was younger, I had a tendency to blame a lot of things on my parents and on my family. But now I recognize that I wouldn't be the person I am today if all those earlier things hadn't happened to me. And I actually really like myself. So, at this point in my life, I find myself in a good place. I feel like I have had the best life."

Midlife teaches us that we can do hard things. We can live through really tough experiences and somehow manage to come out the other side, and what we learn about ourselves in those times can be both surprising and reassuring.

Sadie, who is in her mid-fifties, has a new-found appreciation of her own resourcefulness as a result of dealing with her daughter's ongoing mental health challenges: "I've learned that I have greater depths of personal resources than I thought I did. I keep thinking, 'That's it. I can't take this anymore. I can't do this anymore.' And yet I do. I come up with new approaches and new ways to replenish."

Paige, who is simultaneously dealing with the breakup of her marriage and a pandemic-related job loss, takes comfort in the fact that she can continue to draw upon the strategies that have worked well for her in the past. At fifty-two, she's learned that, in order to move forward in times of uncertainty, she needs to start by slowing down: "I've learned that I need to sink into that slower, stiller space—a place where I can find sanctuary." Because it's not just a place of quiet. It's also a place of strength. "You develop this inner strength that comes from knowing that you can trust yourself. And that's huge."

Alana, forty-three, has also come to recognize that everything she's learned in the past can serve as a resource to carry forward into the future. While she's quick to emphasize that she's led a pretty charmed life, all things considered, it hasn't been a life entirely without struggle. "I've had a beautiful and fortunate life. I'm not going to pretend it's been dramatic and difficult. It really hasn't. But, at the same time, I don't want to lose sight of some of the hard lessons that I did learn, whether it was a tough job choice, the end of my common-law marriage, or attempting to date in my late thirties." She's focused on enjoying her life right now while also laying the groundwork for the future. "I'm trying to make decisions right now that will set me up for a good next decade or two. I'm a little obsessed with that, I think. But I also recognize that I didn't get to forty-three as a happy, useful, generally content human being without making some fairly explicit choices back in my thirties. And so I'm carrying that forward as I begin to think about what my fifties and sixties might look like."

Looking forward

As Deb, fifty-one, continues to map out her own path forward into the future, she's becoming increasingly clear about what she wants and needs in terms of quality of life. She's resisting the cultural pressure to be endlessly productive by making a conscious effort to set aside time to do things she genuinely enjoys. "Doing things for myself—things that I actually enjoy—used to feel like an unnecessary indulgence," she explains. "But at this point in my life, I'm starting to see that it's not. Doing things that I enjoy is what allows me to live, not just exist. And so I planted a vegetable garden in my backyard for the first time this year. I've started painting. I've started writing a novel. These are all things that I love to do and I'm finally giving myself permission to do them."

Susan, forty-five, is also in the process of making those same kinds of life choices but, in her case, instead of adding new activities to the mix, she's starting to let go of activities that have lost their sparkle for her. When we spoke, she was trying to figure out a way to break it to the other members of her choir that she'd made a decision to leave after twenty-five years. It's not that she doesn't love the choir. "It's a wonderful choir and, for the longest time, I thought it would always be part of my life," she says. It's more a matter of wanting to create space in her life for other activities that are more energizing and fun for her right now, like going to concerts and planning small-scale adventures with friends (the only scale of adventure that was possible at the time of our interview, which was smack dab in the middle of the pandemic).

Jean, fifty-three, is less focused on the specific mix of activities she needs in her life right now and more focused on how she wants to feel—and, for her, that means having ongoing opportunities to learn and grow: "Change is key to happiness for me. It's the fire stoking my life. And I need it for that fire to stay hot."

Veronica shares that same sense of forward motion—that desire to keep building on the forty-six years' worth of living she now has under her belt. For her, midlife has been a time of asking herself a lot of increasingly pointed questions about where she's been and where she wants to go: "Over the past few years, I've been having conversations with myself about where I am, where I want to go and where I've been. Just taking the time to do that kind of assessment. And it's not like I'm ready to stop. I have energy. I have enthusiasm. I still have a lot of things I want to do. So the question for me right now is, 'How am I going to get there?'"

For Joanna, the view from midlife is a view that spans out in all directions. In addition to remembering who she was and appreciating who she is, she's also anticipating the person she looks forward to becoming. "I see midlife as a power-up stage—a time to get ready for that next stage of life where maybe you're a little less needed by other people. This is why I'm working toward my master's degree—because that's about the future, and it's something just for me."

The older she gets, the more intentional she becomes about the way she chooses to spend her time. To encourage herself to always be trying new things, she keeps a running list of first-time experiences. She explains: "It sounds kind of foolish, but I was inspired by this story I heard about this woman who decided, as she was turning fifty, that she was going to do fifty things she had never done before. Some of those things were really big things. And some of those things were really small things. It turns out she had never taken a bubble bath. Anyway, I was forty-four when I heard that story and I loved the idea so much that I decided to start doing the same thing too. So, this year, for example—the year I turned forty-six—I committed to doing forty-six new things I've never done before. I keep a list, like a big nerd, and I'm always so excited when I get to add to that list. You see, for me, it's not just fun; it's also very philosophical. I think, as we age, that there's some sort of expectation that we're going to do fewer and fewer things that are new—that we're comfortable with the way our lives are. And yet I feel quite the opposite about it. There's so much that we haven't seen and done yet, even at midlife, and our time is so limited. How can we waste a moment of that time?"

PART II

Body

A Midlife Owner's Manual

— CHAPTER 7 —

The Truth about Menopause

A nnie found herself with so many questions about perimenopause that she ended up setting up a Facebook group with a friend in an attempt to find answers. The forty-five-year-old mother of two teenagers, who has a mid-level corporate job, wanted to figure out if the problematic symptoms she was experiencing (menstrual changes, exhaustion and difficulty concentrating) were, in fact, related to perimenopause and, if so, how she was supposed to deal with them: "Do I seek medical attention for this? Do I change my eating habits? Or is this just something that I have to live through?" she wondered.

She was also looking for more information about the perimenopausal experience in general, information that would round out her understanding of what actually happened as your body moved through this hormonal transition. "It's something that really no one had talked to me about. And so the symptoms I was experiencing seemed to come out of nowhere until someone suggested that maybe they were related to perimenopause."

Up until that time, she'd had a very different conception of how the menopause transition was likely to play out: "You're plodding along. Everything is normal. And then at some point, your periods stop and you have hot flashes for a bit, and then that's it. I knew there was this thing called menopause, which I thought was supposed to happen over a period of about a year, but I didn't realize that there could be an entire decade of changes leading up to that."

The group proved to be a valuable source of information. One of the most important things she learned is that everyone's journey through menopause is unique. She's endlessly surprised by the range of experiences that women in the group share, and the fact that, no matter what kind of seemingly obscure symptom ends up being discussed, there's sure to be someone else in the group ready to chime with a validating "Yeah, that's a problem for me too."

It's hardly surprising that so many women end up approaching menopause from a place of either confusion or dread. Many who have experienced it either don't want to talk about menopause at all or are eager to bombard you with cautionary tales about the hell that awaits you in the not-so-distant future. The cultural silence can be deafening. And as for the horror stories? They can be pretty brutal too. Consider this particularly dramatic example of what I've come to think of as the "you need to be scared to be prepared" school of menopause writing.

This is from Marina Benjamin's menopause memoir *The Middlepause: On Life After Youth*: "Every note struck in the land of menopause feels discordant," she writes. "In fact, the whole thing is like some fairground House of Horrors experience, the only consolation being that once all the ghouls have been sprung on you, and the canned evil laughter has faded, you are delivered at the end of your bumpy ride into an existence of such blandness and monotony (if you believe the rumours) that you almost miss the drama."

So, that's encouraging . . .

It's pretty clear that we're desperately in need of alternatives to the silence and the horror stories. We need honest and frank conversations between friends and across generations—and conversations that start early, so that you're every bit as prepared for the onset of perimenopause as you were for the onset of puberty.

And that's where I'm headed with this chapter: to a place where we can speak frankly, openly and unapologetically about this midlife rite of passage for anyone who has ovaries. (Menopause isn't just a midlife woman thing, after all; it's also experienced by non-binary people and by transgender men with ovaries. But because the focus of this book is on midlife people who identify as women, I'll mainly be looking at menopause through that lens.)

A few basic facts

Before we get into the cultural aspects of menopause, let's start with a quick crash course on the biology. After all, it's pretty hard to talk about women's experiences of menopause without first nailing down a few basic facts and definitions.

So first things first: a couple of key definitions. The term "menopause" is used to describe the phase of your life after your menstrual cycles have stopped. More specifically, you're considered to be "in menopause" or "menopausal" once you've gone a full year without having a period. But menopause is just the final step in a much lengthier process known as the menopause transition, more commonly referred to these days as perimenopause ("around menopause"). Basically, menopause is the destination and perimenopause is the journey (a journey that lasts six to eight years on average, according to the Society of Obstetricians and Gynaecologists of Canada). And as for the timing of the journey? According to the SOGC, the vast majority of women (95 percent of us, in fact) can expect to arrive at menopause sometime between the ages of forty-five and fifty-five, with the average age being fifty-one.

In terms of what you can expect as your body passes through this time of hormonal transition, the answer is a definitive "It depends!" Some women experience a lot of symptoms—periods that are irregular in terms of their timing and their length or the heaviness of their flow, hot flashes of varying intensity and duration, vaginal dryness, mood swings, trouble sleeping—as the hormonal production of their ovaries begins to wind down, while others experience virtually no symptoms at all. It's the ultimate "your mileage may vary" kind of biological experience: roughly three-quarters of women experience some symptoms (though only one-quarter experience symptoms that are actually significant enough to have an impact on their quality of life), and one-quarter breeze through menopause without noticing as much as a single symptom.

And if you happen to be someone who is experiencing a lot of symptoms, here are some encouraging words: most women find that their symptoms tend to be worse during perimenopause than they are after they have passed through menopause, when the hormonal roller-coaster ride tends to settle down. Because, as it turns out, it's a hormonal imbalance that's responsible for most of the misery, with the ovaries ramping down their production of progesterone and then estrogen. As you get closer to menopause—or find your way to the other side—your symptoms become less severe. But even that's not an across-the-board rule. While most women find that their symptoms tend to decrease and then cease within a year of having their final period, some women continue to experience symptoms for years after entering menopause—up to twenty years, in fact, according to Deborah M. Merrill, author of *Mastering Menopause: Women's Voices on Taking Charge of the Change*. (Fingers crossed that you don't end up being one of those symptom outliers.)

So what can you do to minimize menopausal symptoms, if they do end up being a problem for you? The SOGC suggests paying attention to the standard lifestyle fundamentals (healthy diet, active lifestyle, minimizing stress—by this point in your life, you know the drill) as well as limiting your consumption of alcohol, cigarettes and caffeine. They also note that hormone therapy can be helpful in situations where symptoms are particularly severe and where a woman's personal medical history indicates that she'd be a good candidate for this particular treatment. As they explain in their current menopause tip sheet, hormone therapy is generally considered to be a safe and effective way to treat moderate to severe symptoms of menopause (hot flashes, night sweats, mood swings, insomnia, difficulty concentrating and vaginal dryness, for example).

Concerned about the safety of hormone therapy? Here's what you need to know. While the evidence indicates that it's a relatively safe option for most healthy women (according to the SOGC, the benefits of hormone therapy outweigh the risks for "healthy women who start [hormone therapy] within the first ten years of menopause onset"), women who opt for hormone therapy are generally advised these days to "use estrogen/progesterone in the smallest doses possible over a short period of time to address only extreme [symptoms]," according to Merrill. Hormone therapy isn't necessarily an option for every woman who is having a really tough time, so it's also reassuring to know that certain types of antidepressants and antiseizure medications have also proven to be quite effective in managing menopausal symptoms.

And that brings me to the most reassuring menopausal fact of all: menopause is simply not a big deal for the vast majority of women. Researchers analyzing data from the Seattle Midlife Women's Health Study found that just five percent of women described menopause as the most challenging aspect of their lives—this despite the fact that eighty-five percent of women who were surveyed reported experiencing at least one menopausal symptom. The conclusion of this group of researchers? It would appear that "the stressful nature of the menopausal transition has been over-emphasized."

It's worth noting that theirs is not an isolated opinion. As Patricia Cohen notes in her book *In Our Prime: The Invention of Middle Age*, the researchers involved in none other than the landmark Midlife in the United States study reached a similar conclusion. That highly respected group of researchers found that while just two percent of women reported feeling "only regret" when their periods stopped, nearly sixty-two percent reported feeling "only relief." Which kind of begs the question, if menopause isn't actually that big a deal for the majority of women, why do so many of us expect it to be a really rough ride?

Why there's so much misinformation and fear

I suppose the simple answer is that we can blame it on Western culture. As sociologist Sharon Wray noted in an article in the *Journal of Aging Studies*, menopause is a cultural construct—meaning that it's experienced in a particular way in a particular culture and at a particular moment in time. It's a point historian Susan P. Mattern makes in her meticulously researched and thought-provoking book *The Slow Moon Climbs: The Science, History, and Meaning of Menopause*: "The symptoms experienced by women going through menopause are real in every sense. But society has had a hand in constructing them for us." Over the past half-century, there's been a marked shift from treating menopause as a natural part of the life course to treating it as a nightmare chapter in our lives, when we're completely at the mercy of our hormones, and therefore in desperate need of medical intervention, a point that Deborah M. Merrill makes in her book.

Shay, forty-eight, has watched this phenomenon play out in her own life: "A couple of years ago, almost every woman I know was dealing with the physical changes of middle age, but was not really willing to name it. They were going to the doctor because they were feeling depressed or whatever. And so we've turned this into a health condition when, in fact, it is a natural developmental stage of life that we enter into. And if we're prepared for it—if we can acknowledge it—we can face it."

Most who decry the medicalization of menopause are not objecting to the idea that hormone therapy is available. It can literally be lifesaving for women whose lives have been upended by extreme symptoms. What they're objecting to is the idea that a menopausal body is, by definition, a body that demands fixing—a body that's crying out for restoration to its estrogen-fuelled reproductive glory days. In other words, what they're objecting to is the kind of estrogen deficiency framing that journalist Marina Benjamin resorts to in her menopause memoir *The Middlepause* when she describes hormone therapy as "a bridging loan . . . extended to cover debt"—a temporary fix to rely on until you're ready "to face up to the fact that the deficit is real."

The negative framing around menopause spills over into attitudes toward middle-aged women, and in a way that feels really conscious and deliberate. Menopause becomes a tool for social control—a way to erase women at a time in their lives when they might otherwise recognize their power and begin to dismantle the status quo.

So the way that menopause is constructed in our culture has a major role to play in how we experience it in our bodies and in our lives. As Darcey Steinke puts it so brilliantly in her must-read menopause memoir *Flash Count Diary: Menopause and the Vindication of Natural Life*, "It is not menopause itself that is the problem but menopause as it's experienced under patriarchy."

Of course, *not* talking about something like menopause can have a very real impact on our lives as well. Because if we're not being subjected to horror stories about menopause, we're being given the message that menopause is something shameful we shouldn't be talking about at all. It's a cultural silence that even plays out in families. "For a lot of women, it was a hush-hush thing, if anyone in their families was even willing to acknowledge menopause at all. And when there's a void, we fill it with so many negative, scary thoughts," says Ariel Dalfen, a psychiatrist at Mount Sinai Hospital in Toronto.

The media sometimes fills that void in ways that fuel the fear. I'm thinking, for example, of something I read in a recent article in the *New York Times*, a comment that enraged me at the time and that I haven't been able to stop thinking about ever since. The article was written at the point in the pandemic when people were being exceptionally open about the fact that they were showering less often, and the reporter ended up quoting the owner of a hair salon about this supposed trend. That led the salon owner to volunteer some really misogynistic thoughts about "smells" during menopause and, in her opinion, the need to shower twice a day if you're a woman going through menopause.

The antidote to that kind of misogyny and misinformation is accurate information that's not overly medicalized or too scary, the kind of insider information that tends to emerge through frank conversations with other women.

Not every woman has easy access to these kinds of conversations. Research by sociologists Anne E. Barrett and Erica L. Toothman found, for example, that Black women were more likely to discuss their experiences of menopause with friends and family than white women who, in the absence of these kinds of heart-to-heart conversations, tended to rely on medical information instead—a strategy that exposed them to what Barrett and Toothman describe as an overly medicalized model of menopause that only served to fuel their anxiety about aging.

Some women miss out on these kinds of conversations for other reasons. Tricia's mother died at the age of forty-five, so Tricia, who is now fifty herself, has missed out on the opportunity to learn from her mother's midlife experiences. This feels to Tricia like a major loss, not being able to draw upon that first-hand account of a woman going through midlife, "because she really was that sort of barometer for me."

Alana, fifty-two, can relate to those feelings of loss, but, in her case, the circumstances are quite different. "I don't have a relationship with my mother," she explains. "I haven't had a relationship with her since I was thirteen. She's quite mentally ill. And for those of us who do not have a mother to model ourselves on, to ask the questions, to light the path forward, it's really a very lonely and scary experience to go through. And it's not the same as having friends to talk to about it."

The timing of menopause can also be an issue, as Jackie, fifty-seven, discovered when she found herself heading into early menopause twenty years ago. She was just thirty-seven at the time, and her two young sons were just five and nine. She remembers this as an incredibly lonely time: "I had no support. I think everyone around me was shocked. No one could relate to what I was experiencing."

So frank conversations about menopause are anything but universal. In fact, they're still surprisingly rare. And Lisa, forty-nine, wishes they were a whole lot less rare: "I had a great group of women to talk with about childbirth. I want the same sort of openness about menopause."

Julia is also craving that same kind of openness. She wonders why we're willing to be so much more open about puberty than we are about what she calls "reverse puberty"—the hormonal shifting of gears that is menopause. "I have a teenage daughter who is going through puberty. I gave her books to read, and we talk about what she's experiencing and what might help to make her feel more comfortable. We have a framework for dealing with this stuff. And I feel like those of us who are going through menopause need that same kind of framework. There really needs to be a manual and we really need to be talking about this stuff more."

Because when we do find a way to make those conversations happen, they can feel nothing short of magical—a chance to tap into insider information about "the secret life stage that people just don't want to talk about," as Sarah puts it. The thirty-nine-year-old is just taking her first tentative steps into this hormonal land of in-between, but already she feels incredibly lucky to be able to tap into the wisdom of slightly older friends. "I'm so glad that I'm the youngest of my group of friends because these women in their late forties give me all the dirt. It's like being a teenager and having an older sister to go to. I feel like we're back in high school again, where you would compare notes with your friends about your periods and stuff. 'Hey, did you experience this?'"

What women talk about when they talk about menopause

Being able to compare notes with other women can save you a lot of worry and help you find answers to your biggest questions. Questions like, "Is this perimenopause?" and "Is this normal or something that I should be worrying about?"

That first question can be surprisingly hard to answer, which may help to explain how it ended up inspiring the brilliant all-female comedy troupe behind *Baroness von Sketch Show* to create a sketch about perimenopause. "Maybe it's perimenopause," one of the characters muses, only to second-guess herself moments later: "It can't be—is it?"

If you've lived through or are living through perimenopause, you can no doubt relate. Not only is there a huge variation in terms of symptoms, but those symptoms end up morphing and changing over time. And because it can be challenging to get a handle on what you're dealing with right now (as opposed to what you were dealing with last month or what you might be dealing with next month), you can find yourself grappling with that second question quite often too.

It can be really reassuring to know that you're not the only person dealing with a frustrating or puzzling symptom, like menstrual bleeding that has either gone AWOL or haywire. Because of the lingering cultural taboo around talking about menstrual bleeding, many women suffer (and worry) in silence about the often-dramatic menstrual changes that can be part of the perimenopausal experience. As the authors of *Our Bodies, Ourselves: Menopause* note, "The hormonal ups and downs of perimenopause can be the cause of almost any imaginable bleeding pattern." At times when estrogen levels are lower, your uterine lining ends up being thinner, resulting in lighter flow or a shorter period. And at times when it's higher (at least relative to the amount of progesterone coursing around your body), you're likely to experience heavier bleeding or a longer period.

Heavier periods? Annie, forty-five, can relate to that. "I remember last year there was one time I had to go to the mall with my daughter to get her a new phone. Partway through the appointment, I could feel the leak happening. And I had changed my tampon just thirty minutes earlier."

Irregular periods? Tricia, fifty, is living that right now. "I'm in my second month of having sort of an unpredictable period and not knowing when exactly it's going to come—and experiencing extreme pain around the time it should have come when it doesn't show up."

Periods that show up more often than usual? Sam, forty-nine, is familiar with that concept: "My cycles are now a maximum of twenty-one days, but often as short as fourteen days. And I've been like that for two or three years. At this point, I should be getting gift baskets of tampons at my door."

When it comes to perimenopausal bleeding, your best bet is to simply expect the unexpected. And to take solace in the fact that the process will end eventually—and hopefully sooner rather than later if you're having a particularly tough time.

Of course, simply waiting for relief may not be an option if your symptoms happen to be extreme, as Lisa's were. The forty-nine-year-old teacher and union activist ended up seeking medical treatment and, eventually, having a hysterectomy. In her case, her garden-variety perimenopausal symptoms were complicated by adenomyosis (a condition in which the lining of the uterus moves into the muscles of the uterus, leading to exceptionally heavy bleeding). Things came to a head when her bleeding was so heavy that she actually ruined a seat on an airplane. "It was a one-hour flight. And I had just changed my tampon and my overnight pad before boarding the plane." She ended up opting for surgery for quality-of-life reasons.

And, speaking of quality of life, no conversation about perimenopause is complete without a discussion of hot flashes. Hot flashes are the most common symptom reported by women who are going through perimenopause, and according to research led by University of Michigan epidemiologist Siobán D. Harlow, women who experience them are at increased risk of experiencing additional symptoms, such as anxiety, depression or sleep disturbances.

Wondering what a hot flash feels like? They can best be described as thunderstorm-like movements of heat that tend to be as intense as they are fleeting. Menopause researcher Ayelet Ziv-Gal and her colleagues describe them as "sudden, transient bursts of heat" that are particularly pronounced in the upper parts of the body, including the arms and face, and that may be accompanied by such symptoms as skin flushing, profuse sweating, chills, palpitations and anxiety.

Suzanne, fifty-four, remembers how surprised she was by the experience of her first hot flash. "I'd heard about hot flashes, but I just thought, you know, you just get a little warm and you just fanned yourself or took off your sweater. Not this boiling heat that made you feel like you were in a rage and needed to lie down on top of the air conditioning vents in the house."

The hormonal changes of perimenopause wreak havoc on the body's temperature regulation system in a way that makes it hard for your body to maintain a steady temperature. It's like having a climate control system in your home that is too sensitive, one that constantly toggles between "too warm" and "too cold." This is why you wake up repeatedly in the middle of the night to kick the blankets off and then pull them back on. Your inner thermostat has gone a bit wonky, so you're having to toggle that temperature control manually.

But before you start to panic about what hell may await you in the Land of Hot Flashes, it's important to understand that while hot flashes are very common (approximately 80 percent of us can expect to experience at least one), only a small percentage of women (roughly 10 to 15 percent) experience hot flashes that are severe enough to interfere with their quality of life.

If your hot flashes are mild and infrequent, you can probably just shrug them off. Or you might rely on a handful of strategies for minimizing their intensity while you wait for them to disappear over time: dressing in layers; minimizing your consumption of caffeine, alcohol, hot beverages and spicy foods; or relying on deep-breathing exercises and other stress management techniques to manage feelings of anxiety.

But if your hot flashes are particularly intense, they can have a devastating impact on your quality of life. A 2018 study by a group of researchers in the UK found, for example, that women who experienced particularly severe hot flashes, especially ones that happened to occur at work, were more likely to leave the workforce.

None of this is surprising to Alana, a fifty-two-year-old mother of three who works in the non-profit sector. "I'm wildly amazed that women remain competitive in the workforce during menopause," she says. "Everybody likes to talk about how disruptive the childbearing years are, and yet I have not seen any sort of acknowledgement of how incredibly challenging it is to stay competitive—or even just to stay *in* the workforce, when you're struggling so hard, both physically and mentally. And I'm not merely thinking of that in terms of the psychological challenges, but also in terms of the brain fog, the memory issues. It's mind-boggling."

Reaching out for support

If you're struggling with these kinds of extreme symptoms, it's important to know that support is available—both from other women and in the form of medical treatment. You don't have to suffer in silence, nor should you feel like your only option is to wait for these symptoms to subside, a process that could potentially take years to play out.

Sometimes it can take time to untangle everything that's going on with your body and to arrive at the combination of strategies and treatments that will deliver relief.

In Kim's case, it took a couple of months to figure out what was triggering the debilitating migraines she started experiencing earlier this year, in her early forties—migraines that were very different from the ones she had experienced in the past. After experiencing double vision and a debilitating headache that wouldn't end, she went to see her doctor. The diagnosis? Cascading migraines. "He explained that this kind of migraine is most common in women between the ages of forty and fifty-five. The thinking is that, as menopause kicks in and your hormones change, the problem will eventually resolve itself. In the meantime, I'm probably going to be dealing with a partial recovery until I hit menopause." She's figuring out how to manage what have been fairly debilitating symptoms with a combination of medication and lifestyle changes. "The double vision is actually relatively rare now. If I've had maybe a few too many days in front of the computer and I'm just getting run down a little bit, then the double vision kicks in, but I can usually repair that with medication and rest."

For Rachel, fifty, who has been living with chronic illness for a very long time, sometimes a bit of medical detective work is in order. "I remember last year, I had been really very, very ill with my ulcerative colitis and I was put on very high-dose prednisone. I was on a very high dose—the highest that I'd ever been on. I had like 'roid rage [an unwelcome side effect of being on prescribed steroids] and I'd wake up all sweaty in the night and I would say to Jason, 'Prednisone or perimenopause?' So it turned out a lot of it was just prednisone, because when I was weaned off that medication again, the bothersome symptoms went away."

Of course, tapping into support doesn't necessarily mean seeking medical treatment. Depending on the types of symptoms you're experiencing and the impact they are having on your life, you may find it just as helpful (and perhaps even more helpful) to compare notes with other women.

These conversations matter, in terms of both providing much-needed reassurance on a personal level and helping to shift the broader cultural narrative, says Sheri, forty-four: "I'm lucky in that I have a really open network of friends. We've shared our journeys of the last ten or fifteen years with respect to pregnancy, fertility, miscarriage losses—opening up a dialogue about our bodies in a way that likely wasn't available to my mother and her friends. I remember the kinds of messages women were given about menopause back at that time. The butt of every joke was some woman having hot flashes. Today talking about the changes that are happening to our bodies isn't nearly as taboo."

The more information we have about those changes, the less anxious we feel about heading into menopause, which is why we need to have this information *before* we have a chance to develop a lot of menopause-related worries. Because here's the thing: most women find the anticipation of menopause to be worse than the actual experience. As Susan P. Mattern noted in her book *The Slow Moon Climbs*, "The views of younger women on this stage of life are more negative than those of women who have been through it." In other words, it's a whole lot less scary when you're looking at it from the vantage point of the rear-view mirror.

That's certainly been Katrina's experience. She's not just happy to be in menopause, she's actively celebrating. "Every year, I have an annual event that I call 'Crone-iversary.' I mark the anniversary of the date when I officially entered menopause, a year after having my final menstrual period. And, sure, my body is still a bit of a mess. I'm still having hot flashes and night sweats. But there's also a lot worth celebrating about being at this stage of life. And so that's what I've chosen to do. I'm celebrating."

CHAPTER 8

Midlife Mental Health

Tricia isn't sure what's going on with her moods, but she knows that something feels really off. "There's this deep sadness that just creeps up on me some days," the fifty-year-old mother of three and non-profit administrator explains. And then there's the loneliness—a soul-deep kind of loneliness that doesn't make any sense to her. "There are times when I just feel so desperately lonely, even when I'm in a room with my family. I'm not sure where any of this comes from, but I know that I don't want to feel this way. And I can't help but wonder if this is somehow related to perimenopause."

As it turns out, there's no simple answer to Tricia's question. Maybe this melancholy cocktail of emotions *is* somehow related to the hormonal upheaval of perimenopause—or maybe it's not. Maybe there's something else going on. It could be that none of this has anything to do with menopause or midlife—and it's possible that those heavy moods have everything to do with both of those things.

And then there's the fact that, by the time you've reached midlife, you've accumulated a lot of life experience, for better and worse. "You're not just suddenly Zen about life because you turned fifty-seven," says Sheila, who works part-time as a university faculty member. "It's more like, 'Oh, shit, I actually *have* to deal with some of this earlier stuff because the coping mechanisms that I relied on for so long simply aren't working anymore.' Trauma piles up—and at some point, you have to deal with that."

Mental health struggles can occur at any life stage, and midlife adults have been having a particularly tough time in recent years. A recent study published in the journal *American Psychologist* highlighted the fact that middle-aged adults in affluent nations are more likely to experience sleep problems, severe headaches, difficulty concentrating and alcohol dependence than both younger and older adults, and that midlife is a time of life when rates of depression, anxiety and serious psychological distress tend to peak (particularly for women, individuals who are living on a lower income, and people who identify as 2SLGBTQ+).

Unfortunately, a lot of mainstream conversations about midlife mental health are lacking in nuance. There's a tendency to blame everything on menopause—a misguided assumption that only serves to increase suffering by convincing you that you're supposed to feel this way when that's actually not the case at all. Symptoms of depression and anxiety are neither universal nor inevitable—not for women going through menopause and not for midlife women in general. You don't have to simply settle for feeling miserable.

Figuring out what's going on

A crucial first step is to really pay attention to how you're feeling. How does your current mood compare with your usual mood? Is this something new or different—perhaps something more intense? And how long have you been feeling this way? Is this a transient emotional cloud that is just passing through or a more persistent emotional storm that has been hanging around for weeks, months or even years? And then, once you've actually acknowledged what you're feeling, you can start trying to figure out why—what seems to be fuelling all this heaviness and misery.

Ariel Dalfen, a psychiatrist at Mount Sinai Hospital in Toronto, has had a lot of experience in guiding women through the process of trying to figure out what isn't working. The goal of this inner detective work? To identify the problem so that it then becomes possible to find solutions. "Maybe you're depressed because of some life changes that have been happening—all those midlife identity shifts. Maybe you're depressed because you're experiencing some physical symptoms that are interfering with your sleep and your functioning. I would really want to focus on answering the question, 'What's causing this?'"

And while she rejects the idea that hormonal changes are the root cause of all midlife misery, she is quick to acknowledge that hormonal shifts *can* be a major problem for a small group of midlife women. "We know that certain women are very sensitive to hormonal fluctuations at all life stages. These are women who—when their estrogen and progesterone levels fluctuate around the time of their period or during pregnancy, postpartum, or during menopause—do develop significant psychiatric symptoms. But that's not everybody. And in most people, there is some other contributing factor. So women shouldn't just assume that because your body is going through all these changes—and because you're at this particular life stage—you're inevitably going to be depressed. That's not the case at all."

Sometimes midlife mood swings can catch you off guard, even if you're someone, like Tamara, who is exceptionally tuned in to her own mental health. (She's a psychologist as well as the mother of seven-year-old twins.) "What I didn't really factor in on a more personal level, as opposed to an abstract level, were the hormonal changes," she explains. "Especially if you became a mom a little later in life like I did (I had my twins at age thirty-seven), sometimes you just don't pick up on everything that's going on. You have all of the hormonal shifts that happen after having your children; and then, if you're an older parent, it's not too long after that that your body starts throwing you an entirely new set of curveballs. I remember thinking when I had my first hot flash, 'How is this possible? I just finished with postpartum hormones. I feel like I finally got to a stable place and now I get thrown this thing?'

"I think it's very hard as a woman to recognize that so much of your mood—so much of how you move through this world—can be dictated by something that's out of your control. That hormonal shift has been a wallop for sure. And it just feels like such a kick in the ass for so many women. You spend your life trying to manage your hormones and figure this stuff out, from the time you're a prepubescent girl and then all the way through pregnancy, birth and postpartum. And then you find yourself recognizing, as you head into perimenopause, 'Okay, now I have to deal with this too.'"

And that's assuming, of course, that you even know that perimenopause is a thing, she adds. "A lot of women say, 'I didn't even realize it was happening' because they certainly weren't expecting any sort of hormonal shift to be happening quite yet. They had that long view of menopause. And unless you have some really overt symptoms, you don't always put them together to recognize what's happening."

And then, of course, there's the wildcard that is stress. Not only do menopausal symptoms increase stress, but stress can worsen menopausal symptoms. You might need some support in breaking free of this nasty cycle.

Knowing when to reach out for support

It took Sandra, a fifty-year-old freelance communications consultant, a while to notice and acknowledge, even to herself, just how terrible she was feeling. Her symptoms kicked in the summer she started her own business—a challenging situation that became immeasurably more challenging after she fell and broke her elbow and wrist. Add to that the fact that she had started to experience some sort of hormonal shift ("I started feeling really low, particularly in the lead-up to my period") and you can see why she quickly found herself in a pretty bad place, particularly since she was convinced that this was something she should be able to handle on her own. "I deeply resisted the idea of talking to anyone about it. After all, what did I have to feel down about? I lead what many would call a privileged lifestyle. I am married to my high school sweetheart whom I still adore, I have two kids who are pretty great, and I make decent money working for myself. Complain? Why? Also, it was very clear to me that the 'low' feeling really showed itself at very specific times in the month, and it was not a constant thing."

The situation deteriorated until it reached the point where it was clear that she needed to get off this "mental health roller coaster." That's when she turned to her doctor for help. She tried following his initial suggestions—that she try an antidepressant and speak to a counsellor—but those suggestions didn't offer any relief. "Things got worse, and I went back, and this time the doctor suggested going on the pill, as I knew the low times were tied to hormones somehow. I went back on the pill, but four months later, developed a blood clot, which meant I had to stop taking it." In the end, she was referred to a women's health clinic at a major hospital—a place where she finally felt seen and heard. "They were wonderful, taking the time to really understand what was happening with me. Hormone testing revealed that I was right: my estrogen was basically non-existent in the weeks leading to my period, which was definitely contributing to feelings of depression. Unfortunately, due to the blood clot, I was not eligible for hormone replacement, which they believed could have helped me greatly. So again, I was back to square one, in terms of treatment options"—an antidepressant combined with various lifestyle modifications.

Sandra finds it frustrating that midlife mental health continues to be shrouded in so much mystery: "I feel like this stage of women's health is not well understood, and there are not enough options to help women through this. It is tremendously disappointing and frustrating. And it's only through the network of other women that you find out about what could possibly help. A close friend is the one who told me about the clinic that I found helpful, and I had to ask to be referred there." And while the clinic wasn't able to offer any magical solutions, "At least at the clinic, I felt heard."

Alana has found herself on a similar quest for answers and solutions, but, in her case, the mental health challenges that she's been dealing with at midlife aren't new. In her case, they're more like a variation on an old, familiar theme, the fifty-two-year-old mother of three and non-profit administrator explains: "I have a history of depression that's complicated by both a history of trauma and a history of hormonally driven physical issues. I've been struggling with premenstrual dysphoric disorder since I was a teenager, but my symptoms became much more extreme when I entered perimenopause."

Her initial attempts to obtain treatment for what she was experiencing proved to be an exercise in frustration. "There was no attempt at contextualizing or considering the interplay between my various issues. What I encountered instead was sort of an either/or approach. Either you are experiencing some sort of mental health crisis, or this is something that we can just throw some medication at and call it a day. But there was no attempt to dive in and figure it out."

It wasn't until she managed to get an appointment with a women's health specialist that she finally got the comprehensive workup she needed—one that endeavoured to put all the puzzle pieces together. "This was the first time that a medical professional took the time to dig into my health history, to do a full blood workup, and to really consider the social context of what I was experiencing too. My forties had been just a haze of crises."

And that's when things finally started to get better for Alana. The workup was comprehensive enough to pinpoint the fact that her symptoms are cyclical: they ebb and flow along with her hormones. "I have two weeks when I feel okay, and then the anxiety and other symptoms really start to ramp up before I end up hitting a crescendo in the two weeks prior to my period," she explains. Pinpointing that pattern made it possible to identify strategies for minimizing the intensity of her mood swings. "The doctor told me, 'You have a condition that is manageable, but you also need to look at your life-style and your stressors, because you're going to have to find a way to live with this. What can you do in your life to alleviate some of the stress that you experience in the two weeks of your cycle when your symptoms are most acute?' It was such a relief to be talking to someone who wasn't in a hurry to write me a prescription for yet another antidepressant or to send me away with a fistful of Ativan. This was someone who was actually willing to work to find a way to support me."

Weathering the storm

Having the right health professional to support you through times of struggle is key. But how do you go about finding the right person?

You might want to start out by asking your family doctor for recommendations—assuming, of course, that you're lucky enough to have a family doctor and you have a good relationship with that person. You might also consider comparing notes with other women you know who've weathered these kinds of struggles themselves and who were fortunate enough to find a supportive mental health professional. Of course, all this assumes that you actually have the luxury of choice—that you live in an area where it's possible to find a mental health professional who is taking on new clients, and that you have the ability to pay any fees that may be required. That's not necessarily a given for all women. In fact, it's a major challenge for many.

But assuming that you do have options, you'll want to think about whether the particular mental health professional you are considering feels like the right person for you. "Look for someone who is going to listen to you, who's empathetic, and with whom you have a good connection," suggests psychiatrist Ariel Dalfen. "And don't feel like you have to settle for the first person you see. If the two of you aren't on the same wavelength, keep looking for someone else."

Paige, fifty-two, knows from first-hand experience just how important it is to be able to turn to a health professional you trust when you're weathering the storm of a mental health crisis. She recalls how deeply she was struggling at the time of her bipolar diagnosis twelve years ago and what a critical role her family doctor played in guiding her to a place of wellness: "The diagnosis was a bit of a shock. No one in my family had ever been diagnosed with any mental illnesses, so it felt strange and out of the blue for me. And I remember that first year vividly. I was experiencing a really deep clinical depression along with an especially gripping kind of anxiety that was triggered by one of my medications. And I remember feeling like my life was over—that I was never going to find a way through this. I was really on the edge, and I was even having intrusive thoughts about ending my life. But there are moments when the universe sends you that little piece of hope—and, for me, that hope came in the form of my GP, who's just an amazing doctor. I told her how much I was struggling, and she said, 'Okay, here's the thing. We just need to get your medications sorted out. I have nearly a hundred patients with bipolar illness and almost all of them go through this process—and we almost always get it sorted out. You are going to have a happy, healthy life and I'm going to help to get you there.' She made me promise to call her every day for the next two weeks and to promise that I wouldn't do anything to harm myself while we sorted the medication issues out. She knew exactly what I needed to hear, and she said it with such compassion. I honestly think she saved my life."

It's so important to hear that kind of message of hope, particularly if you're really struggling or if you're new to a particular mental health diagnosis, says Dalfen. "You need to know that what you're dealing with right now is just a stage in an illness, a stage where you're beginning to understand what it means to live with this diagnosis. You start to understand your symptoms: what they mean and how you can manage them. You begin to figure out what does—and doesn't—work for you; what things are—and aren't—within your control; and who you can turn to for support. You need to know that it won't always be this hard."

Paige remembers just how hard it was, especially during those really dark days. That's one of the reasons she chooses to speak frankly about her own struggles. She wants other people to know that it's possible to find your way to a much happier place. "There is hope. There are so many people like me who manage to get through this. And they don't just manage to get through this; they actually go on to create a rich and beautiful life for themselves, because they have learned how to treat themselves and others with compassion. Because that's what happens when you make it to the other side: you get to be there for someone else. You get to talk people back from the edge by telling them, 'I once stood there myself.' And that truly is a gift."

— CHAPTER 9 —

Your Body at Midlife

Lori's grasp of the expressive elements of dance has never been better. A couple of decades after she first set foot in a dance studio, the forty-three-year-old former competitive dancer feels like she's on top of her game creatively. She's finally figured out what so many former teachers tried to teach her and what she simply didn't have the life experience to understand until now: tapping into an inner groundswell of emotion turns mere movement into art.

It's exhilarating, but it's also frustrating because the arthritis she's developed in her foot makes it difficult for her to translate that epiphany into movement. "I have a greater understanding of what dance can do. But now that I've figured it out, I can't do it," she says.

While dance will always be part of Lori's life, her days of pursuing a career as a performer in the world of tap, jazz or ballet are definitely a thing of the past.

Sure, she can dance for an hour or two at a time.

She can head to the workout room to "bang out" her frustrations on a tap board if she's having a bad day.

But she can't commit to anything regular or sustained—not if she wants to avoid severe pain or further injury.

And that, for Lori, continues to be the biggest challenge of midlife—coming to terms with these bodily changes. "I'm channelling some of that artistry and self-exploration into other activities, like the fiction writing that I do, which I love. But I still feel that need to let energy out through my body and, in the case of tap, to play with sound as well as movement."

And so, she'll continue to hit the tap board as often as she can—as often as her feet will allow.

Our bodies are constantly changing. It's a process that starts long before we are born and that continues through each stage of our lives.

Back when we were kids, we celebrated these changes, noting with excitement how much taller we were at the start of each school year. But then, at some point, we stopped paying as much attention. The changes were a whole lot more subtle, so it was easy to convince ourselves that our bodies were pretty much staying the same (unless, of course, we happened to sign up for that mind-blowing biological transformation known as pregnancy).

Most of us coasted along like that for a while—maybe even for a couple of decades. Unless we had a specific reason to pay attention to the day-to-day functioning of our bodies (perhaps because we were living with a chronic health condition), it became easier to take our adult bodies for granted, to assume that, with the exception of the odd grey hair, it would likely be business as usual for at least the foreseeable future.

And then everything changed. We arrived at midlife. We swapped the body we had for a very different body—what feminist gerontologist Martha Holstein describes as "an attention-demanding body."

It's pretty much the perfect term, because a midlife body can be pretty good at insisting you pay attention, as Alana has discovered for herself. "Things are creaking, and you're like, *what is that?* I'm only forty-three!" Or, she adds, you start to notice that you're feeling really tired. "You can eat all the kale you want and you're still going to be a little more tired than you used to be at eight o'clock at night, after putting in a full day."

Leigh, forty-seven, has been picking up on some of these midlife body changes too: "It starts with creaky knees, maybe. Or a few grey hairs. Then, a few years later, you're throwing your back out after lifting a house plant!"

So you've officially arrived at the point in your life when you can no longer ignore the fact that you have a body. Slowly but surely, your body begins to shout, "Pay attention!" in ways that you can no longer ignore. As narrative gerontologist Molly Andrews pointed out in a recent article, this is one of the lessons that we can't help but learn as we grow older—the fact that we are "embodied selves."

And that's what we'll be talking about in this chapter: how to truly embody midlife; how to give your body what it needs, in a loving and non-punitive way. Your body, like the rest of you, continues to be a glorious work-in-progress.

Stress and the midlife body

You'll notice that I didn't include the word "self-care" in the title of this chapter, nor did I splash it on the cover of this book. That was an intentional decision on my part, in recognition of the fact that a growing number of midlife women are practically allergic to the term. And how could they not be, given the narrow, high-pressure and guilt-inducing way it tends to be framed these days, especially on social media?

Instead of being rooted in ideas of self-compassion and the need to safeguard the precious resource that is you, self-care has devolved into something much more superficial and commercial—a meaning-less and often expensive quick fix when what your body is screaming out for is something resembling actual care. This, of course, is the very thing Audre Lorde was getting at when she wrote about the radical political implications of practising self-care—of preserving herself in a world that was hostile to her very existence as a Black woman. For her, self-care was much more about "self-preservation" than "self-indulgence."

In the absence of that powerful, political framing, self-care simply becomes something else to feel guilty about. Either you feel guilty for taking that time for yourself when you could be taking care of others or doing something productive, or you feel guilty for *not* being able to take that time.

For Lara—who describes herself as a forty-seven-year-old military wife, mother (to an atypical teen), teacher, Indigenous person (Secwépemc–Métis) and survivor (of both PTSD and the Sixties Scoop)—the guilt of not having time for self-care is accompanied by a layer of worry about what the future holds for her body. "I worry about fragile bones, and maintaining my ability to move. I worry about moving from middle-aged to old and what that will look like. I worry about my heart, my health, my muscles, my blood pressure, my bones. I don't ever want to be frail, but I know the pressures of life right now too often prevent me from taking care of myself as I should. We're told that we are supposed to take care of ourselves so that we can take care of others. That thought is exhausting. How do I do this when there are so many demands on me? I always feel as if I'm short-changing myself. We only live once. Am I messing it up?"

Simplistic self-care messages ignore the complexity of life for midlife women, and it's hardly surprising that a growing number of women reject them. Eileen, forty-two, feels like those messages miss the mark, and miss the mark badly: "Almost every piece of advice I come across says to take time for yourself, the buzzword being 'self-care.' Which, I'm sure, would be very helpful if I could actually do it." Self-care is easier said than done "if you're home with young children, your family is incapable of helping or too far away to help, there are no babysitters, your spouse works a lot, and then, heaven forbid, a pandemic cuts you off from any school time or hired help of any kind," she explains. Even something apparently simple like taking a bath can feel frustratingly unattainable: "Alone? When? When you're up from dawn to dark with kids, dealing with their online schooling, keeping them from fighting when you're on a call or otherwise working from home, and fielding calls from nurses about your elderly parent, there often isn't enough time to rest, or exercise, or read a good book—at least not alone."

Like Eileen, Alex wholeheartedly rejects the idea that self-care platitudes and simplistic solutions are adequate ways to address the challenges facing midlife women. "The idea that the self-care that women want is a bubble bath and a pedicure? *No!*" A psychologist in her mid-forties who also happens to be a single parent, Alex isn't willing to settle for anything less than systemic solutions that actually address the heavy load that so many women like her are carrying. "We want someone to share the load, we want our boundaries respected, we want social structures in place to help us continue with having careers," she explains. And she wants women to radically redefine the concept of self-care, both for themselves and for others. She longs for conversations that dig deep into this issue. "I want to be able to ask other women, 'What's sustaining you through midlife? What practices or rituals do you find helpful?' Because the load is really heavy."

A critical first step in that project of redefining would involve actually acknowledging the weight of the load so many midlife women are carrying. Clearly, there's a need for more and better research on this front. As a group of nursing researchers from Seattle University and the University of Washington noted in a recent article for the medical journal *Midlife Women's Health*, the original tool that was designed to measure stress was developed with the lives and experiences of male naval shipyard personnel in mind. As a result, experiences that women would consider stressful simply didn't show up on the list of potentially stressful life events. Even today, these tools aren't great at measuring what stress looks and feels like for women in general, and for midlife women in particular. That's why the researchers highlighted the need for studies that offer insight into how stress experiences change over time as women go through menopause, and that take into account the fact that midlife women often find themselves dealing with "multiple co-occurring stressors" that have a tendency to snowball over time (a job loss that leads to financial pressures that trigger a relationship crisis, for example). In other words, there's a need for research that actually acknowledges the complex ways that stress plays out in the lives and experiences of middle-aged women.

At this point in her life, Angela would settle for something as simple as a basic acknowledgement that stress is, in fact, an issue. The forty-eight-year-old author and university lecturer is still furious about the way stress was consistently omitted from the conversations she had with her former family doctor over the years about her various health concerns. She recently obtained a copy of her medical records and was shocked to see how often "diet and exercise consultation" appeared in isolation, without any mention of the underlying factors that might be triggering symptoms such as stress eating. "We'd be having a conversation about my weight or my cholesterol or whatever but there was never, ever any acknowledgement of all the stress I was under." And, as it turns out, Angela's stress load was massive and unrelenting. "When my son was a newborn, I had postpartum depression. Then we supported my mother through a decade of cancer treatment, while simultaneously raising a young child. And when my mother moved into a hospice, we took over the care of my grandmother, who was living with dementia and Alzheimer's. And then, of course, I was dealing with my own physical and mental health issues at the same time."

Angela was dealing with a lot—and yet her former family doctor never even thought to ask her about how she was doing. If he had, maybe he would have been able to connect the dots between the heavy emotional load she was carrying and the physical and mental health symptoms that kept bringing her back to his office. And by not asking that question, he silently telegraphed a powerful message—that Angela should be able to handle all this stuff on her own.

It's a message that a lot of midlife women hear and internalize: stress is simply a fact of life and it's up to you to figure out how to live with it. And that's a major problem, as sociologists Nancy Mandell, Susannah Wilson and Ann Duffy point out in their book *Connection, Compromise, and Control: Canadian Women Discuss Midlife*: "Because we accept that stress is an individual's responsibility to manage, there are few structural supports to relieve it."

And, boy, could we use some relief, especially during those times in our lives when the whole concept of "self-care" feels impossibly out of reach.

That pretty much describes Jude's relationship with self-care for many years: it just wasn't happening. It *couldn't* happen, in fact. During this time, Jude—a non-binary agender person in their early forties—was so deeply immersed in meeting their child's needs that they simply didn't have any additional capacity to take good care of themselves. "When I was parenting, I was so exhausted, I couldn't imagine walking any farther than the two blocks it took to get to the library. I was forever in survival/crisis mode, just trying to make it through another day from the time the alarm clock went off (necessitating twelve attempts to wake my son up to go to school) until bedtime (when I would have to confiscate his smartphone to keep him from being online all night)." It wasn't until Jude's son made the decision to live with his other parent—a painful and devastating decision for Jude—that Jude was finally able to prioritize their own health. "There are two hard truths I hold: I love and miss my son. But I would not be enjoying the life I am living now if he hadn't left," they explain.

That extra bit of breathing room, painful as it was, has given Jude the capacity to start focusing on their own health. "I had been diagnosed with diabetes about nine months after my son moved out. That meant I had to completely change what I was putting in my body. And I finally accepted the fact that I have been living with c-PTSD [complex post-traumatic stress disorder] for all these years and started really focusing on therapy for myself (as opposed to merely arranging therapy for my child)."

Jude has also been working on their relationship with themselves: "I like to think about, 'Who am I to myself?' As a result of spending so many years taking care of other people (my family of origin, my former husband, my child), I forgot that I'm a person that also deserves that much support and that I need to make it happen. That has meant prioritizing myself and learning to ask for help from friends. I care less about what other people think of me, and more about what I think of me. I'm working on self-compassion and rebuilding the self-esteem that got crushed both when I was a young teenager and then later, every time I was told I was a bad mother."

Beyond self-care

Sometimes the most powerful and life-changing thing you can do is to simply start treating yourself with more compassion: to change the channel in your brain from self-critical to self-compassionate, and to start seeing yourself as someone who is worthy of care.

It's an approach to wellness that resonates with Indigenous Elder Jo-Anne Gottfriedson, sixty-nine, who is a member of the Tk'emlúps te Secwèpemc people in the Interior of what is now known as British Columbia. "In my culture—and especially within my family—we are taught from the moment we are born that we are sacred, that we should honour ourselves, and that we must take care of ourselves," she explains. "I think women need to rekindle that self-worth and look at themselves as beautiful and worthy and sacred."

And when you start to see yourself that way, you want to treat yourself that way. Starting from a place of self-compassion makes it easier for you to be kind to yourself, even if you aren't managing to meet the guilt-inducing self-care standards set by everything from social media checklists to the ideals of your younger, less busy self. Take Angie's situation, for example. These days, the forty-eight-year-old writer, editor and mother of two, is not nearly as active as she used to be. "I spent most of my life as a runner, biker and so on," she explains. "And I'm not doing any of those things these days. But I'm finding different ways to be active. We've had a 'no car in town' rule for a decade and I've always done a fair bit of walking over the course of a typical day. So my definition of what constitutes exercise has changed." Treating herself with self-compassion means focusing on what's reasonable and possible for her right now, while also recognizing that what her body needs from her will continue to evolve over time. "My body is showing more signs of wear and tear. My hips and back are a lot more vulnerable. So I'm not sure I'll go back to running, and I certainly won't be doing marathons or half-marathons anymore. I'm thinking that walking and yoga are better bets for me, once I have a bit more time. Because I really don't have any time for myself right now. And while this means I'm probably exercising far less than I ever have at any other time in my entire life, I just keep telling myself, 'This is okay for now. It won't be this way forever.'"

Self-compassion is deeply rooted in that message of acceptance—acceptance of what is (and isn't) within your control, even if you don't love the situation. Instead of beating yourself up about what isn't possible, you shift your focus to embracing what is.

For Claire, a forty-year-old mother of two and the founder of a non-profit organization, that means paying attention to the health fundamentals that help her to stay well: "I take care of myself like it's a job because I'm susceptible to anxiety and depression. I focus on the preventative approach of eating well, exercise and rest. These used to be things that I pushed aside in the past, but now they are necessary to my day-to-day."

Sometimes it's a life crisis that transports you to this place of self-compassion—that suddenly shines a spotlight on the need for actual, meaningful self-care. In the aftermath of her brother's death earlier this year, Paige, fifty-two, has been doing a lot of thinking about the kinds of health changes she may need to make for the sake of her own well-being: "When you experience the death of a sibling, as opposed to a parent, there's this heightened sense of mortality. You begin to appreciate on a really personal level that there are no guarantees in life. My brother was just ten years older than I am. He was very young in passing. And his death left me with a lingering sense of *this could be me*, as well as a lot of questions. If I only have a decade left, what do I want to do with that time? And if I do have the opportunity to have more time, what kinds of changes do I need to commit to, because it's pretty clear that some pretty extreme self-care needs to happen."

Danielle can relate to those feelings of anxiety—plus an intense desire to do anything she can to stay healthy. The forty-seven-year-old mother of two, who with her husband runs a general contracting company, has spent many decades of her life living in the shadow of her mother's death—wondering if she, too, was destined to leave her young daughters motherless at an early age. "For me, it wasn't a matter of wondering if I was going to get cancer, but when," she explains. And then it happened: Danielle was diagnosed with colon cancer while undergoing some unrelated screening tests during a period of ill health. Fortunately, Danielle responded well to treatment, at least in part because her cancer was detected early— so early that she describes her diagnosis as "a gift." Her only regret? "That my mother didn't have that same chance."

Practising self-compassion has the potential to shake up your world in far-reaching ways. While the changes you make may prove to be the right ones in the long run, they can be really tough to work through in the moment, as Lisa discovered.

The forty-four-year-old queer mother, anti-violence educator, activist and researcher realized, at the peak of the pandemic, that she had to make some significant life changes in order to prevent her health from spiralling any further downward. Not only does she live with an inherited connective disorder called hypermobile Ehlers-Danlos syndrome that is complicated by other health conditions, including high blood pressure, but she's also been carrying a heavy load on the family and career fronts, too, trying to meet the needs of her two children, who inherited the same disability, while also devoting her career to "high-stakes, nonprofit, anti-violence work."

Recently, she recognized that something had to give because she was paying the price with her own health. "The work I do is work that really makes a difference in the world. But, in caring for others, it has been really hard to care for myself. And I think at this point in my mid-forties, I'm recognizing that I only have so much time left and that I have to start prioritizing my body and my health. It was very, very hard for me to finally admit to myself and other people, 'I can't do this job anymore. It is killing me. I am sick, in the middle of a pandemic. I need to take care of myself, and I need to create room in my life to actually have fun.' When I shared my decision at work, people were shocked. They kept saying, 'What are you thinking? You're at the top of your game.' And they were right. I am at the top of my game. But I told them the same thing that I've always said to my kids, something that I truly believe: the time to leave a party is when the party is at its height—when you're having the very best time and before things get ugly. In terms of work, I stayed a minute too long, but in the end, I listened to my body. I decided that it was time to go, to do something different and to use my gifts in a different way."

Shelly has also been making some far-reaching life changes aimed at supporting her own wellness and quality of life. The forty-nine-year-old mother and grandmother who is employed as a writer, college instructor and retail worker, explains: "About five years ago, my husband and I sold our family home, which we had lived in for more than twenty years. We moved into an apartment in the city core. We were trying to move to a simpler, less complicated lifestyle, a smaller lifestyle that had a little bit less to do with stuff. At this point in my life, I want to be able to visit my children and grandchildren in other parts of the province for a couple of weeks at a time. Being in an apartment makes it so much easier to do that. We just shut the door and off we go. So that was a lot of it. But then there was also the issue of where I choose to spend my energy. When you have depression, your energy tends to be unpredictable. And when the energy is good, I want to be able to use the energy doing things that make me happy rather than doing all the things that have to get done when you're taking care of a house."

What a body needs

Finding a way to give yourself the space you need to think, to breathe, to be—that may very well be the most powerful form of self-care. It opens the door to considering what your mind and body actually need, in order for you to feel and function at your best.

For many midlife women, sleep is at the top of that list: sleep is the glue that holds everything else together. When we're getting enough sleep, we feel calmer and happier. We find it easier to concentrate and we're more likely to have the energy to be physically active (which, in turn, encourages good sleep). Okay, that's the good news. Now the bad news: at midlife, sleep tends to be in chronically short supply, with generally high stress levels and bothersome menopausal symptoms like night sweats conspiring to rob us of the rest we so desperately need. Whether it's because we struggle to fall asleep or to stay asleep, most of us end up falling short of the seven to nine hours of sleep our bodies crave. According to a 2017 data brief published by the U.S.-based National Center for Health Statistics, 59 percent of perimenopausal women and 40 percent of postmenopausal women report sleeping fewer than seven hours, on average, in a twenty-four-hour period. Is it any wonder that so many midlife women feel like they're sleepwalking through their lives some days?

Feeling chronically exhausted can also interfere with even the best intentions to be physically active—even if you know in your heart that engaging in regular physical activity will actually boost your energy level and help you to sleep better at night. It's one thing to know that on an intellectual level; it's quite another thing to convince yourself to get back up off the couch when it just feels so good to close your eyes . . . And, of course, a so-called lack of motivation is only a tiny slice of the pie chart explaining why so many women are less active than they'd like to be. Research led by University of Washington health researcher Kathleen Smith-DiJulio points the finger of blame at the patriarchy—or, more specifically, the impact of gender roles. Her research revealed that women often feel like they have to focus on meeting other people's needs first, which means that their own health needs end up being put on hold. And, what's more, a recent study published in the medical journal *Midlife Women's Health* identified time constraints, economic pressures and safety concerns as barriers to women's physical activity. So what we're talking about isn't a matter of individual willpower and motivation; it's something much bigger and nastier than that. When only about half of midlife women are able to meet the current physical activity guidelines for aerobic activity and only one-quarter are able to meet the guidelines for muscle strengthening activities, something is seriously wrong and in need of fixing.

Giving our bodies and minds what they actually want and need often means resisting the pressure to be endlessly busy and productive.

This is something that Kat, a forty-three-year-old white woman and disabled mother of two, has been thinking about a lot. This thinking was sparked by some of the learning and unlearning she's been doing in response to some of the teachings of the Black Lives Matter movement, "looking at white supremacy as the root of all things capitalism—the valuation and the commodification of the human body. We're taught that we need to perform, we need to be active, and we can't rest. It was really shocking to me to realize that a lot of my inner thinking was actually institutional framework, messages I'd absorbed from the broader culture." That realization led her to start paying attention to a tendency in herself to turn to productivity as a coping mechanism, as a means of pushing through feelings of grief about some of the losses she's experienced in her life. "For me, it became a really toxic cycle. If I was having trouble sleeping, I'd get out of bed and work. It was my way of trying to compensate for other areas of my life where I felt I was falling short of my impossibly high expectations for myself. Being productive is so valued in our society. We're told we have to keep going—we have to keep doing. But at some point, I recognized that this wasn't working, and I said to myself, 'Hey, Kat, you know what? You need to stop everything and just unplug and rest. The solution here is *not doing*.'"

It's a message that so many of us need to hear: You don't have to demonstrate your worthiness by forcing yourself to be endlessly productive. You are a person who is worthy of care and rest. And as for proving yourself? You honestly have nothing left to prove.

Consider these wise words from Sheri, a forty-four-year-old mother of three who works in government: "Just being a woman who has a lot on the go, and who is okay for whatever reason—that in and of itself, I think, is quite radical."

In other words, just being okay is a pretty big deal. It's enough.

Confronting health-related worries

Here's a rather worrisome statistic: the vast majority of midlife women are anxious about aging and about declining health in particular. According to sociologists Anne E. Barrett and Erica L. Toothman, who have studied women's anxieties about aging, the thing midlife women worry about the most is declining health. Only one in five midlife women actually manage to steer clear of this particular worry.

It's not surprising that so many of us are carrying this particular worry around. We receive so many cultural messages telling us that aging well is all about making good choices, that it's our own personal responsibility to "age well," which basically means not becoming a "burden" to anyone else. It's a simplistic and wrong-headed narrative— and one that causes a lot of unnecessary worry and even fear. As J. Brooks Bouson notes in *Shame and the Aging Woman: Confronting and Resisting Ageism in Contemporary Women's Writings,* "The chronically ill, disabled, and physically infirm elderly become receptacles of the projected social fears of dependency, vulnerability, and failure that lurk just below the surface of our competitive, success-driven and individualistic culture."

This narrative not only fuels a lot of unnecessary anxiety but can actually increase the likelihood that we'll end up in poorer health. There's a solid body of research to show that people who treat declining health as inevitable and unstoppable are less likely to seek treatment for their health problems. And that, in turn, can actually lead to a shorter life. A 2002 study led by Yale University epidemiologist Becca R. Levy found that older adults who have negative views about old age tend to die seven-and-a-half years sooner than their peers. In other words, this kind of toxic, life-limiting thinking has a measurable impact. Ageism doesn't just harm; it kills.

What we're talking about here is basically ageism directed at the self, with a hefty side dish of ableism thrown in. It's a toxic combination that erases the experiences of a lot of women and that conveniently sidesteps the structural factors that are in play. A healthier approach would be to recognize disability as "an essential element of human diversity represented by at least 20 percent of the general population at any given point in time"—and even more of us as we grow older—*and* to acknowledge both the inequities that contribute to these differences and the supports and structural changes that might help to prevent or mitigate them, in the words of disability studies researchers Clara W. Berridge and Marty Martinson.

Unfortunately, Alana, fifty-two, is picking up a lot of those ageist and ableist messages in her conversations with other midlife women. The non-profit administrator and mother of three describes it as an almost tangible fear—and one that the wellness industry is only too happy to capitalize on: "I think there's just so much fear about cognitive decline. People are terrified to even consider the possibility that they're not 100 percent on their game. And the number of women that I've talked to who have embraced that fiercely ageist 'successful aging' thing is astounding. They honestly believe that if they work hard enough at prioritizing their wellness, they will somehow manage to 'defy aging.'"

It can be helpful to acknowledge what's at the root of these fears. For some people, it's the mistaken belief that "it's all downhill from here," an oversimplistic narrative of decline that erases the fact that midlife and beyond are times of both losses and gains. And for others, it's a fear of being dependent on other people.

Let's start with the first worry—the idea that all you have to look forward to from now on is decline. It might be helpful to consider the changes that have been happening to your brain, just as an example of how this narrative is anything but true. Sure, you may have lost a bit of processing speed over the years, but your older and wiser midlife brain can leave your younger brain in the dust when it comes to making connections, spotting patterns and building bridges. And if you're worried about that loss of processing speed, it's worth remembering that what's measurable in the laboratory doesn't necessarily translate into a noticeable difference in day-to-day functioning. This nuanced reality is the same for your other organs and body systems.

Now on to the next worry, the fear of being dependent on other people—of struggling to get your needs met in a culture that celebrates independence rather than dependence and that punishes people for not measuring up to that anything-but-reasonable standard. The more you unpack this belief—the idea that we expect people to be completely autonomous in terms of their care needs as they age—the more ridiculous it becomes. For starters, it's not an expectation we carry over into other life stages. Do we insist that newborn babies be self-sufficient from the moment they are born? No, we do not. Nor is it an expectation that we carry over into other areas of our lives. Are we expected to build our hospitals and highways on our own, or do we find ways to create this physical infrastructure together? The answer is obvious once again. But when it comes to providing care or investing in care infrastructure, we suddenly back away from that collective approach to problem solving, choosing to treat aging and dependency as problems that individuals and families are required to solve on their own.

And what's different about this care work, of course, is that it is overwhelmingly work that is performed by women, either within our own families or for often subsistence wages in the wider economy. This systemic failure causes huge suffering for women: not only are we more likely to live with chronic illness or disability as we age, but we're also more likely to be providing care to others. Yes, I'm standing on my soapbox and I'm shouting, and I'll have a lot more to say about this in the final few chapters of this book (you *had* to know I wasn't done talking about this yet!), but for now I'll simply say this: we need to consistently and loudly challenge the narrative that says that aging well means aging on your own. Because here's the thing: it's a narrative that only works well for men, plus a handful of truly privileged women (women who either win the health lottery or who have the financial resources required to get their own care needs met). We need to insist on a very different narrative, one that celebrates interdependence, not independence.

Tapping into some disability wisdom

So now that we've tackled those two gigantic worries, I want to focus on something much more positive and reassuring. I want you to know that it's possible to live well in an aging body. In fact, it's more than possible; it's the norm. You see, we humans are amazingly adaptive. We have the ability to come up with wildly creative solutions to really challenging problems. People in the disability justice movement have coined the term "disability wisdom" to describe the tremendous resourcefulness of disabled people when it comes to adapting, innovating and just plain reimagining their lives. You'll probably feel a whole lot less anxious about facing bodily changes as you grow older if you reject any limiting, ableist ideas about what that might mean. Instead of assuming that your quality of life will be compromised, you might find it tremendously reassuring to choose instead to learn more about how disabled people feel about themselves and their lives—"how they discover and make meaning in the world," as public health researcher Susanne Schnell put it in a recent article in *Generations*.

And that's why I want to wrap up this chapter by tapping into the wisdom of people who have been living with chronic illness or disability for a very long time.

People like Rachel, Karen and Andrea.

When I ask Rachel, a fifty-year-old mother of two, to describe herself, she cuts right to the chase: "I guess I'm just going to start with the fact that I'm chronically ill. I don't like that fact to define me, but it's a very big part of my life. I'm chronically ill. I have a very rare liver disease called primary sclerosing cholangitis and I stopped working ten years ago because of my health. Before that, I was working a full-time job and raising little kids. It was exhausting. Of course, that stage of life is exhausting anyway, so it's hard to say how much my liver disease contributed, but I started finding myself in this downward spiral. I kept getting infections and I'd end up in hospital four or five times each year. And then my liver started to fail. That happened when I was thirty-seven. After that, I managed to find a living donor and I ended up having a liver transplant. My thinking at that time was that, in about a year, I'd be going back to work, and everything would be fine. Well, everything *wasn't* fine. I tried going back to work on two separate occasions, but I just couldn't do it.

"It took me a long time to accept that my life wasn't going to be the same because my body wasn't exactly the same as it was before. And by saying that it took a long time, I mean that I'm still grappling with that realization right to this day. Even now, it's really hard for me to actually say to myself, 'I'll never work outside the home again.' Like, that's it!

"I've really worked hard to try to find joy, and to try not to just be wrapped up in guilt or in feeling sorry for myself. Don't get me wrong: I feel sorry for myself all the time. I have issues with this whole 'heroism of illness' thing. You don't have to be a hero. You just have to figure out your day-to-day. While that doesn't seem like very profound advice, taking that approach has really helped. Because you just can't plan too far in advance if you have a chronic illness."

For her, that's meant learning to accept the fact that she's going to have good days as well as bad days, and that when she's having one of those bad days, one of the kindest things she can do for herself is to find a way to go with the flow. Often those moments of struggle happen in the middle of the night, when she finds herself wide awake despite the fact that her body desperately needs sleep. "One of the side effects of the immunosuppressants I take is chronic insomnia. When I first started dealing with this, I would get really anxious about the fact that I was having trouble falling asleep. But over time I've learned to simply acknowledge and talk myself through this situation. I'll say to myself, 'Since I'm wide awake, I'm just going to read. If I fall asleep, that's great; if I don't, that's okay too. I don't have anything pressing I have to do tomorrow.'"

If there's an upside to living with a chronic illness (and Rachel is the last person who would insist that anyone has to find an upside), it's the fact that she's forced on a daily basis to consider where she wants to invest her energies and what does—and doesn't—work for her. She quickly discovered, for example, that she's not a great traveller. "A couple of times we tried to take trips, but I ended up in bed in a hotel room for a couple of days, trying to recover from the flight." Better bets for her are simple activities that she can incorporate into daily living, like having dinner as a family and playing board games together. "I may not have what some people might consider a quote-unquote *normal* or *typical* life, but, for me, it's a pretty great life."

Like Rachel, Karen wishes that able-bodied people had a greater understanding of what it's actually like to live with a disability: your life isn't perfect, and your life isn't terrible—it's somewhere in the middle, just like everyone else's. She also wishes that they'd ditch a lot of other really ableist assumptions—either underestimating what she's capable of or judging her for not being able to do more. "Able-bodied people do that all the time. They think that, if you have a disability, you are incapable of everything else. It isn't until they are forced to be up close and personal with someone with a disability that they realize that all of their assumptions were incorrect. I also wish they would stop assuming that they're in a position to judge what I am, or am not, capable of, because people do that all the time."

If people weren't quite so quick to rush to judgment, they'd quickly see that Karen, who lives with severe and debilitating chronic pain, has a strong sense of meaning and purpose. This is not to in any way diminish the severity of that pain. The fifty-one-year-old, who retired a decade ago for medical reasons, admits that living with chronic pain and intractable migraines has had a major impact on her life: "My time is spent in bed, either reading or watching television. I get out of bed for a few minutes at a time, to make myself a meal or to go to the washroom. And then I head back to bed."

But that's only part of the picture. There are other days—joy-filled days—when she volunteers to transport rescue dogs to their new homes. "I drive rescue dogs because the dogs give me a reason to stay alive. Cuddling a dog alleviates a lot of the regular pain that I experience. I'm not feeling that pain right in front of me. It's relegated to a background position. And not only that, but the dogs are incredibly loving, and in a way that so many humans aren't. Spending time with the rescue dogs is so joyful. And for a life that has so much pain, you grab on to joy anywhere you can find it and you hold on. Of course, it's also exhausting. The moment I arrive home from taking these dogs to their new foster homes, I have to take a nap because I'm in pain and I'm tired. But I can get up the next day because I've done that. I have a reason to exist."

Andrea J. Buchanan has also found solace in the company of others, but, in her case, those others have been humans, not canines. Connecting with others who are living with the same chronic illness has taught the forty-nine-year-old writer and mother of two the importance of having strategies for coping with the challenges of daily living. And, in her case, those challenges have been considerable. She was diagnosed with mast cell activation syndrome after experiencing a cerebrospinal fluid leak (a life-upending experience that she documented in her powerful and moving memoir, *The Beginning of Everything: The Year I Lost My Mind and Found Myself*).

"I'm living with a chronic illness and my life is kind of shaped around that," she explains. "And by that, I mean it shapes a lot of the decisions I end up making on a daily basis. Things like, 'I was sitting up for four hours, so I probably need to lie down for two hours, so I can get up again.' That sort of thing. And so finding a community of people who are either dealing with the exact same thing as you are or going through something similar can be hugely helpful. It helps you to feel so much less alone. These people actually understand what you're dealing with because they're living it or have lived it, too, and they have so much valuable information to share. You can turn to them and say, 'Has this happened to you? If so, what did you do?' It feels a lot like early motherhood in a lot of ways. You really need to find your pack."

CHAPTER 10

Body Love

"What does it mean exactly to love your body on its own terms, as it is now?"

Samantha Brennan and Tracy Isaacs pose this question in their book *Fit at Mid-Life: A Feminist Fitness Journey*—and Brennan proceeds to answer in a really powerful way. "What does it mean to 'love' this body? I don't think it's perfect, aesthetically speaking," she writes. "That's not what I mean at all. I could list all its flaws . . . but I won't. I love my kids. I don't think they are perfect. I'm not talking about aesthetics and I'm not talking about perfection. I don't associate either of those values with love."

I've probably read those words a hundred times over the course of the past year, and yet every time I read them, I am transported to a place of radical self-acceptance, a place where my body doesn't have to be anything to be deemed worthy of love. My body can just be. It's a place of freedom, calm and joy—and a place I couldn't have even imagined visiting, back when I was trapped in a decades-long state of self-neglect and self-loathing.

"Body shame flourishes in our world because profit and power depend on it," writes Sonya Renee Taylor, a Black queer author and activist, in *The Body Is Not an Apology: The Power of Radical Self-Love.* A key piece of my own midlife journey has been rejecting body shame and stepping into a place of body love. I am choosing to live my life in a way that robs profit and power of at least some of its body shame supply.

It's not necessarily an easy journey. Not only are we likely to be carrying around a lot of cultural baggage about body image in general, given our culture's toxic and limiting messages about what a body is supposed to be, but now we also get to add a new layer of messaging related to aging. And so, for many of us, midlife becomes a time of recognizing and working through messages of internalized ageism—what psychologist Mary Pipher and others have described as "prejudice against one's own future self."

Sheila, who is fifty-seven, remembers struggling with those feelings, back when she was in her early forties. "I remember looking at women who were maybe ten years older than I was and actually feeling afraid. I remember asking myself, 'Am I going to look like that?' I remember feeling like I wanted to distance myself from these women. And I remember being both deeply aware of my own internalized ageism and very troubled by what I was feeling." Sheila ultimately managed to work through these feelings. A decade later, those friends who are ten years older no longer seem "ancient" to her. But it took time for her to make sense of all the thoughts and feelings that were bundled into that initial visceral reaction to the signs of aging on her friends' faces.

And that's what we're going to be talking about in this chapter: why so many women have such a visceral fear of the physical signs of aging and what we can do to defuse that fear. In other words, we'll be looking at ways of making peace with both the bodies we have and the bodies we will have, so that our journey through midlife ends up being one that is rooted in love, not fear.

Becoming invisible

Who gets to decide who is and isn't visible? The people in power, that's who. And we know who has that power and who it is they'd like to erase. As Mona Eltahawy notes in her brilliant and incredibly validating book *The Seven Necessary Sins for Women and Girls,* "Attention is both reward and punishment. It is how patriarchy regulates us."

It's deeply disconcerting to realize that someone is trying to erase you—and that you're actually being encouraged to erase yourself. As feminist poet and theorist Adrienne Rich noted in an essay published more than thirty years ago, it can feel like you're looking at yourself in a mirror and seeing nothing.

Shay has noticed that this experience hits some women harder than others. The forty-eight-year-old Black woman, who is the executive director of an anti-racism organization, explains: "There's this tendency to erase women, particularly at middle age, and I think that plays out differently across racial lines. All midlife women end up being erased, but a white woman's experience of erasure is different from how I feel erased, because white women are valued for their beauty in our culture. I mean, to some degree, Black women are used to being erased. Black women have always been treated as somewhat invisible, whereas, for white women, midlife might be the first time they've faced that—the first time they've [experienced that devaluing and invisibility first-hand]. I don't always feel like white women are as equipped to deal with midlife. In fact, I think they can get smashed really hard by it."

There's a solid body of research to back up what Shay has been noticing in her own circle of friends. Research conducted by sociologists Anne E. Barrett and Erica L. Toothman has revealed that there's definitely an intersectional element to what they describe as "declining-attractiveness anxiety," with white women being more anxious about declining attractiveness than Black women, and heterosexual women being more anxious than non-heterosexual women about becoming less attractive and losing their reproductive ability. As sociologist Jessie Daniels notes in her brilliant and important book *Nice White Ladies: The Truth about White Supremacy, Our Role in It, and How We Can Help Dismantle It*, white women are highly valued for their role in "reproducing whiteness" by becoming mothers.

Katrina, fifty-one, has watched this play out in her own life as a conventionally attractive heterosexual white woman. "You can go through life as a younger woman being pretty and charming. And you could be *only* pretty and charming and everybody will think you're wonderful because you're pretty and charming. And then you get to be middle-aged and you're not conventionally pretty anymore and not necessarily so charming anymore. Suddenly, you start to lose value—or at least that's what some people would have you believe." It's the price women pay for having so much of their value under patriarchy tied up in rigid beauty norms.

All that said, it's important to keep this issue in perspective. Anxiety about declining attractiveness only tends to be a problem for a relatively small group of women—roughly 10 percent of us, according to Barrett and Toothman. And, as for the increased invisibility that comes with age, many women, including Sheila, greet that with a certain amount of relief. "There's something really joyful about being invisible—of finally being freed of all this shit that we've been dealing with since puberty. Suddenly, it's so quiet when you're out and about, doing your thing. You're not being heckled or harassed in the same way. And that's a really positive thing."

Trish, fifty-five, is also grateful to be dealing with less unwanted attention when she heads out for a walk, but, at the same, she doesn't feel that "the lessening of the male gaze" necessarily has to mean arriving at a place of invisibility. "The sidewalk whistles are light years behind me, thankfully. That kind of attention angered me always," she explains. "But the absence of that kind of attention doesn't make me feel less visible. In many ways I feel more seen and heard at age fifty-five than I have ever been. Yes, there is still a critical gaze for middle-aged women—the pressure to cover your grey hair, to battle that tummy bulge. Comments meant in kindness from long-time friends, like 'you never age' or 'you never change,' as though we're supposed to live in a time capsule. We *do* age and we *do* change, in good ways and in less good ways. I wish we lived in a world where we didn't have to create a fiction around that. There are things I can't do today due to bodily wear and tear, yet there are things I can do today that I'd never imagined or had only dreamed of doing. But somehow, with age, I've become a lot more comfortable in my own skin. And that is such a relief."

Forever young?

Of course, feeling comfortable in your own skin means battling market forces that stand to profit from making you feel insecure about the physical processes of aging. As Patricia Cohen puts it in *In Our Prime: The Invention of Middle Age*, "Activate insecurities about middle age and you create a lifelong customer."

And not only do women feel a lot of pressure to engage in what is known as "age-mediated aesthetic labour"—the work people (mainly women) do to conceal evidence of age—but they also feel deeply conflicted about succumbing to that pressure. It's yet another one of those damned if you do, damned if you don't situations—the patriarchy working its usual magic, in other words.

The decision about whether to dye their hair tends to be particularly fraught for a lot of women, at least according to research led by Vanessa Cecil, a PhD student in psychology at the University of Exeter. Women who choose to continue to dye their hair often worry about "looking fake, inauthentic or [being] subject to disapproval for not being age-appropriate." And yet, at the same time, there's always some random stranger ready to warn you of the dire consequences of not dyeing your hair, like the psychologist who offered what I've come to think of as the worst beauty advice of the pandemic, when she warned the readers of British *Vogue* of the perils of going grey without consulting their partners first: "In extreme cases it could lead to divorce."

Katrina, fifty-one, recalls how difficult it was for her to stop dyeing her hair. "I really struggled with that. I went back and forth a couple of times. I look ten years younger if I dye my hair, and men really discount women who look like they're no longer fertile. I realized that I really missed men hitting on me." At one point the situation got really weird: "A friend of mine was going on a date, and she said, 'This guy wants to bring his friend. Can you just come along as well?' I agreed, and just to have fun, I decided I'd wear a wig." (At this point, her hair was completely grey—and the people she was planning to hang out with were a few years younger than her.) As it turned out, "the friend was super into me. And I did show him what my hair looked like—what I looked like without the wig. He later asked me to go to some function with him but asked if I would wear the wig. And I remember thinking at the time, 'Are you hitting on me or are you hitting on my hair? Why don't I just send you the wig?'"

And just as Katrina resents the weird messages women are given about dyeing their hair, Laura wishes people would lay off on the issue of wrinkles. "Why is it considered shameful if we look like this?" the forty-seven-year-old former radio host asks. "Sixty percent of the lines on my face are from laughing my head off or making other people laugh. These wrinkles have brought a lot of people a lot of joy!"

It seems to me that midlife women would benefit from a whole lot less beauty advice. Carolyn, for one, is pretty fed up with the endless barrage of messages. The forty-nine-year-old mother and health-care worker explains: "I find it strange that there's always this small but really vocal group of people who want to tell women what to do with our lives. And it happens at every life stage. I mean, even at midlife, we're still getting policed. We're being given so many conflicting messages about what we should and shouldn't wear, for example: 'It's okay to wear crazy outfits.' 'You really should dress sexier—or not.' 'You're showing too much cleavage.' 'Don't wear your hair that way!' 'Who do you think you are, wearing those clothes?' No matter what you do, no matter what age you are as a woman, you're always being asked to live up to these impossible societal expectations. The difference is that now I have the confidence to say, 'You know what? I don't care. This is what I want to wear. This is what I'm going to wear. This is my body. Love it or leave it.'"

Making peace with your body

Love it or leave it, indeed. Midlife is a time in our lives when we have an opportunity to make peace with our bodies. Of course, that's often easier said than done, and it's never more challenging than when it comes to the issue of weight. Because if there's one area where we're particularly vulnerable to criticism about our bodies, that's it. A study published in the medical journal *Current Psychiatry Reports* in 2019 found, for example, that nearly three-quarters of midlife women struggle with feelings of dissatisfaction about their weight—and that those concerns can show up in any number of different ways, from generalized concerns about your weight or your shape to full-blown eating disorders.

For some women, it's a long-standing struggle.

Beth can clearly identify the moment in her childhood when she began to fixate on her body—the Valentine's Day when a classmate wrote a particularly cruel poem about her that poked fun at her weight. The fifty-year-old entrepreneur and mother of two teenagers explains: "I remember laughing about it, but that was just a defence mechanism, trying to convince people that I didn't mind being teased. But I did mind. And it did have an impact on me. Throughout my entire adult life, I've been very regimented in terms of what I eat. I beat myself up if I even gain a pound. And I got certified as a personal trainer. You can't help but bring that kind of childhood experience of bullying with you, as much as you can try to get over it. And, as a really overweight kid, I got bullied a lot."

Laura can relate to Beth's experience of looking at the world through a lens of body preoccupation. "How much energy in my brain went to thinking about 'What am I wearing, what do I look like, who's the biggest person in this room? Is it me?'" the forty-seven-year-old muses. "I often wonder where I would be in terms of my relationship with my body right now if I hadn't been sucked into diet culture."

Shauna, fifty-three, has been thinking about that too. She recently found herself flipping through a bunch of photos of herself when she was younger, remembering what it felt like to be that person. "I remember thinking at the time that I was fat, because that was the message I kept getting from my mom. Any discussion about my body seemed to end with her saying, 'Here's a diet book.' And yet when I look at those same photos a couple of decades later, I can't help but think to myself, 'Holy shit: I was hot!' Why was I so worried about how I looked? I wish I could have all that time back. *All that time.*"

For other women, weight and shape concerns are something that didn't show up on their radar until quite recently, after decades of being reasonably happy or even very happy with their bodies. That's how things have played out for Jackie, a fifty-seven-year-old educational consultant and the mother of two young adults. "I had a hysterectomy in my mid-fifties, which changed my body dynamics, energy levels and weight," she explains. "I'm still working through trying to get a handle on the best way to deal with what seems to be a new body shape for me."

And she definitely isn't alone in that struggle. As the authors of a study published in the *New Zealand Journal of Psychology* noted, Western cultural pressures on women to remain thin, regardless of age, are "almost completely at odds" with the biological changes experienced by the majority of midlife women.

For some women, those kinds of biological changes are complicated by other factors. Consider Rachel's situation, for example. The fifty-year-old chronically ill mother lives with a rare liver disease that fluctuates in terms of severity, causing her weight to fluctuate too. "A lot of people comment on my weight—and I don't love it. If I'm weighing more, I'm probably healthier. If I'm very thin, I'm probably pretty sick. It's so problematic in society anyway, but for me, it's like, 'Thanks, but I'm actually feeling well. And also, *just don't comment on my weight ever.*'"

You don't have to be carrying around a lot of extra weight— or even any extra weight at all—to be plagued by these torturous weight-related worries. They're a problem for so-called "normal" weight women too. And frankly, how could that *not* be the case? As the authors of that same study in *Current Psychiatry Reports* noted, by the time they arrive at midlife, some women have devoted decades of their lives worrying about and trying to manage their weight. Why would those weight-related worries magically disappear at a point in their lives when their bodies are actually inclined to *gain* a bit of weight? It's hardly surprising that many women engage in "extreme behaviors to delay the natural signs of aging" and that over half of so-called normal weight women (women with a body mass index that is less than 25) report being less satisfied and more unhappy with their bodies in their fifties, as compared to when they were younger (even in their forties).*

Of course, it doesn't help that women are subjected to so many toxic messages about midlife body changes. These messages are so ubiquitous that they often don't even register in our brains unless they're particularly obnoxious, like this description for a particular line of swimsuits, designed for women over the age of fifty. Martha highlighted this product for me during our interview, describing it as a product that encourages midlife women to "internalize all the body hatred." The company describes itself as being on a mission to "camouflage" the evidence of "a life well lived." And as for what is allegedly in need of camouflaging? What women's magazines used to euphemistically describe as "problem areas." The resulting product is a swim dress that's designed to cover your upper arms and part

---

* Just as an aside: Body mass index (BMI) is a problematic measure at best. Because it's based on height and weight measures alone, it ignores other really important factors like muscle mass, bone density and racial and sexual differences. My goddess weight—the weight at which I feel my best—indicates that I'm overweight. I considered editing out the BMI reference but I decided to leave it in, because BMI is the measure that these particular researchers used. But that doesn't mean that I love it. No, dear reader, I do not love it at all.

PART III

Soul

On Navigating Change and Finding Community

CHAPTER 11

Midlife Epiphanies and Curveballs

Susan has been doing a lot of thinking about what she actually wants for herself. Recently, the forty-five-year-old life coach and writer has been noticing a strong feeling of inner restlessness—an overwhelming desire to make big changes in her life.

"I have been feeling the same way that I felt back when I was in high school, which was that the world is exciting and full of possibility, and I am not getting any part of it. So much of being a teenager involves having this strong sense of anticipation and suspended possibility—you're just going through the motions in your daily life while looking forward to a time when you can get out there and live your real life. And that's exactly how I'm feeling right now: I can't wait to finish up this part of my life so that I can get on with the next thing—the thing that I actually want to be doing."

And as for what that thing might be, she's still figuring it out, but she knows it will have something to do with adventure. "I had always thought that we would be the kind of family that had adventures together. But my husband's not an adventurer, so that just kind of got left by the wayside," she explains. And she recognizes that change isn't practical or even possible for her right now. While she feels a little trapped within the confines of "this typical mom, suburban Stepford kind of life," she refuses to do "the other stereotypical

I agree with Jean. A lot of people do need to hear that message—and I think it's something we need to spend more time talking about. Without those conversations, it's easy to assume that everyone else is doing new and exciting things and that we're pretty much failing at midlife if we're not working hard at improving ourselves. Do we really need to invent another life stage that's all about endlessly critiquing ourselves and pushing ourselves to be "better" in some simplistic, self-help kind of way? No, we do not.

It's a lot to think about, for sure, but I think it's definitely worth talking about: where these sky-high expectations come from, who benefits from making us feel like we're doing midlife wrong if we're not committed to some bootcamp-like program of self-improvement and reinvention, and how we can liberate ourselves from these rather soul-crushing ways of thinking.

So, sure, let's continue to learn and grow, but let's do so in a way that's life-enhancing, not stress-enhancing, and that's more about opening ourselves up than tearing ourselves apart. Because maybe—just maybe—the change we're craving is something much bigger than anything that can be tackled at the individual level. What if it's less about wanting something different and better for ourselves and more about wanting things to be better for all of us—to be given the gift of witnessing significant progress in our lifetimes? I'll have a lot more to say about this in the final chapters of this book, but I just wanted to plant this tiny little seed for now, to get you thinking about the rather insidious ways that these one-size-fits-all midlife cultural narratives can really mess with your head, and to remind you that you can choose to push back.

Midlife epiphanies

Not content to settle for things the way they are? Hey, join the club! Midlife can be a time of restlessness—the kind of restlessness that can open the door to new possibilities as you dare to admit to yourself, perhaps for the very first time, that the status quo isn't working for you (or it isn't working for you anymore).

The past year of Kim's life has been about opening new doors—literally. The fifty-year-old non-profit administrator and mother of two is newly divorced, living in a new neighbourhood and starting to map out a new path to the future. She has a strong sense of being at a crossroads as she surveys the landscape of her life. "It's a time of beginnings and endings. The ending of being a full-time caregiver to children, the winding down of a career, and the opportunity to craft a new life, all about me, in the future. It's scary and exciting."

The far-reaching upheaval of the pandemic has encouraged Angela to start thinking about what is—and isn't—working in her life as well. She still hasn't figured out all the answers, but at least she's been able to pinpoint the key question: do I really want to be working this hard? The forty-eight-year-old university lecturer, author and mother explains: "My husband Paul and I have been making some decisions about how much each of us wants to be working. We've been asking ourselves questions like, What do we actually need? What are we actually working so hard for—a retirement that's still twenty years away? And, do we honestly want to sacrifice the good health we have right now? Of course, we want to save for the future, but we've started considering whether, in fact, we might have been focusing on that a little too much, and at the cost of missing out on time that we could be spending with our son. We only have one child. He's fourteen and he still loves to spend time with us. But I imagine that, five years from now, he'll be off pursuing his own adventures.

And so maybe we need to be taking better advantage of the time that we have with him right now."

Being brave enough to ask yourself these kinds of tough questions makes it possible to imagine something better. And that *something* doesn't necessarily have to be something huge—nor does it have to be something that you commit to doing right now.

Jill's decision to leave her job as a partner in a veterinary practice wasn't one she arrived at quickly or easily. The forty-five-year-old mother of three simply started paying attention to the voice inside her head that kept telling her that she was no longer happy with her job. "I told myself, 'It's okay to stop doing this at some point, if you need to'— and, for a while, that really sustained me. It helped me to feel that each day I was going to work by choice, not because I had to." Eventually, she decided to take a bit of a gamble—to leave her job without having another job lined up right away. It's a gamble that ultimately paid off. After taking a few months off, she landed a job as a researcher in the public service. "It's very different from private practice, but I'm really enjoying it. In fact, it's really reinvigorating me, by reminding me about everything I love about being a veterinarian."

As Jill discovered, it can be a huge relief to suddenly recognize that you have options. Instead of feeling trapped in the confines of your own life, you find a way to create a bit of emotional wiggle room for yourself. "What makes it powerful is the choosing," explains Sara Smeaton, a certified coach who specializes in working with people at midlife. "Whether it's a small choice or a big choice, the fact that you're the one choosing it is what makes it powerful. And if that choice is tiny, it's tiny."

Of course, sometimes the change that you know you need to make is anything but tiny. Sometimes you feel compelled to make a change, even though it feels uncomfortable or even scary, because *not* making a change feels even worse.

Sam remembers reaching that tipping point, around the time of her fortieth birthday. That's when she decided to leave her marriage and to come out as gay. "I'm someone who knew they were gay from a very young age," the forty-nine-year-old birth worker and mother explains. "But I grew up in a small town. My dad owned his own business, and I was explicitly told, 'You're not allowed to do anything that might give him a bad reputation.' I was expected to do the right thing—with the right thing meaning that I was expected to get married and have children. Which I did. Unfortunately, it was an abusive relationship that lasted far longer than it needed to. But finally, as I was approaching forty, I thought to myself, 'I'm done. I can't live in an abusive relationship anymore. But, more than that, I can't live with someone who's not the person I'm supposed to be with. And I don't know who that person is that I'm supposed to be with, but it's pretty clear it's not supposed to be a man.' It was a matter of telling myself, 'This is who you are and now you need to honour that.' And that was huge for me."

It's incredibly liberating to be able to step into that place of integrity. Because, as Kathleen A. Brehony notes in her book *Awakening at Midlife: A Guide to Reviving Your Spirit, Recreating Your Life, and Returning to Your Truest Self*, there's a price to be paid for not being able to honour your own truth: "Conforming to social expectations and to a persona that doesn't adequately reflect our deep inner self is like going through life wearing shoes that are too tight: . . . you can walk . . . but you can't dance. And at midlife, the soul is demanding to dance."

It wasn't until her marriage was ending that Jacki, who is now in her late forties, recognized that she had been forcing herself to wear the wrong pair of shoes. "Sometimes you don't realize the discomfort that you're living with until you actually try on a pair that feels amazing," she recalls. In her case, that better-fitting pair of shoes was consensual non-monogamy. "I remember thinking, as my marriage was ending, 'I don't know if I ever want to be monogamous again.' I decided that I wanted to pursue relationships where my partners and I had the freedom to allow connections to form wherever they might and to see where those connections might go, where there wouldn't be any need to stifle a spark that I bring out in them or them in me." And that's the way she's been living her life for the better part of a decade, in a happily non-monogamous relationship with a committed long-term partner.

For Jacki, midlife has been "a time of being open to possibilities and not having to confine myself to a mould." Her advice to other women who may be questioning the rules that seem to govern their life? Don't be afraid to feel whatever it is you're feeling. "There's definitely a lot to think about when you're making these kinds of life decisions, but there's a reason why you've got that little voice in your head telling you to pay attention. Find a way to give space to that voice. Try not to ignore it because these kinds of things don't just go away. And know that we don't have to necessarily give up these parts of ourselves. There are ways to make things work. We don't always have to follow the 'rules.'"

Katrina, fifty-one, recently decided to rewrite the rules of her own life, heading back to school to study psychotherapy. "The rules that we think exist aren't real. They're just societal constructs that we've accepted. But they don't have to be true," she insists.

Two years ago, she figured out a way to ease out of some of the obligations in her life so that she could head to Europe for a couple of months. "I handed my apartment over to my daughter and her boyfriend, along with the keys to my car." What made her escape possible was her new-found ability and willingness to take chances in a way that simply wouldn't have been possible back when she was younger. "I realized I didn't have to play it safe anymore. Both my kids had moved out. No one was depending on me. And so I quit my job."

A critical first step was simply paying attention to what she actually wanted and needed. "I needed to be completely unencumbered. I needed to be in a completely different place, a place where nobody knew me and where I didn't have any bills or any kids. I just wanted to get away from it all. I wanted to be able to wake up in the morning and say to myself, 'I have no idea what I'm going to do today.' I wanted to have the chance to do all the things I hadn't been able to do when I was younger because I'd gotten married and had kids. And so I headed off to Europe without a plan, just like some crazy seventeen-year-old. I did it for the sake of my own well-being and it was great."

Junia was also motivated by her own well-being when she made the decision to come out as a transgender woman. It was a decision that cost her her job as a pastor at a suburban Baptist church. She understood those risks going in but decided it was worth it. Sure, she had a lot to lose, but she also had so much to gain.

"Transition in midlife is almost always really disruptive. It can cost you relationships, it can cost you your career, and it can bring all kinds of unwelcome stigma and instability into your life. There aren't many of us who make this decision lightly. You don't really have any choice as to whether you're transgender or not. That's just the way you are. But you do have some options when it comes to transitioning, and there are trans folks who never transition. Not everyone has the option of transitioning. And while there are people who are able to announce that they're transgender without a lot of upheaval, for a lot of us it's not that way. So we have to be savvy about it."

For Junia, that meant proceeding slowly as she moved from quietly questioning her gender identity in conversations with her therapist and a select group of trusted people to making the decision to transition and to actively present as female in the world. At some point, something shifted. She remembers thinking to herself, "June, you're not dressing up like a woman. You're dressing up like yourself. You're presenting your authentic self to the world. And you need to start making plans to make this happen." And for her it was a year of "training wheels, baby steps" as she began to chart a course toward her new life—getting to know the person she always was and sharing that person with the world.

Midlife curveballs

It's one thing to hit the eject button on your life. It's quite another to have life hit the eject button for you. But sometimes unexpected events force you to grapple with the big questions of life.

Alex found herself grappling with those kinds of questions in the aftermath of her father's death. "A year ago, my dad had a stroke and then he died," the psychologist, academic and single mother in her mid-forties explains. "He didn't have a partner and I don't have siblings, so I had to go back to Quebec for about a month and hold his hand until he died. And then I had to get all of his affairs in order. The experience of watching one of my parents die really made me think about my own mortality. Death has always been a real big part of my thinking, but there's something about your parent dying that makes you think about it even more. You realize, 'I'm the next generation up. I've got a finite amount of time. How do I want to spend that time?' I remember being twenty and just feeling like the whole world, everything, was possible. And I don't feel that anymore at all."

For Beth, it was the shock and shame of being downsized that triggered this same kind of soul-searching. "That was a really tough pill to swallow, to be honest with you," the fifty-year-old entrepreneur and mother of two explains. "At that point, I'd been with the company for seventeen years. I'd started at entry level and worked my way up to the director level. I felt like I had my entire life mapped out. We were a financially comfortable dual-income household, the kids were doing well, and then—boom! Honestly, I didn't see it coming. I had been working in HR, so I knew that there were challenges within the organization, but you never think it's going to happen to you, that you're the one who is going to be laid off."

But then it happened, and Beth found herself reeling. "I remember thinking, 'What do you mean I'm being laid off? I've been loyal to the company all these years and now you suddenly decide you don't need me?'" She was also forced to face the stigma that often accompanies job loss, even if you've been downsized. "I honestly didn't know what to tell people. Imagine having to tell your parents that you basically just got fired. It was a really awkward conversation." One of the hardest things for Beth was the loss of routine and identity that she experienced during the early months, while she was still trying to figure out what to do next. "I didn't have a routine. I felt very lost. I wasn't even sure who I was, given that I wasn't this corporate director anymore. I hadn't realized how much weight I had put into that job title, how much of my identity was tied to being a leader." She eventually emerged from this crisis with a new sense of purpose. She decided to launch her own HR consulting firm. But for a while, it was rough. "I had to work through all these different emotions."

Joanne's midlife curveball came in the form of a sexual assault at work. She had been working as a nurse on a family health team in a small town, a job that she loved because it allowed her to establish long-term relationships of trust with patients. But then that trust was shattered. "I was sexually assaulted by a fifty-four-year-old male patient as I was administering a memory test in a tiny exam room," she recalls. "It was the strangest experience for me, as a strong and confident woman. I scolded him immediately for grabbing at my breasts and trying to pull me toward him. He apologized, but then he did it again. I managed to escape from the room and to get back to my desk, where I proceeded to chart the incident." It wasn't until a day or two later that the experience really started to sink in, and Joanne realized that she needed to take some time off to do some thinking. With the support of a therapist, she came to realize that nursing no longer felt like the right choice for her. "It started to feel like a scratchy woollen sweater that was a size too small." She had already been thinking about different ways she might be able to use her education and experience to support mothers. She was not only a former labour and delivery nurse but had also been through times of struggle in her own early motherhood days, as someone who found herself "married, divorced and a single mom with two kids living on welfare by the age of twenty-three." The experience of being sexually assaulted on the job accelerated that thinking. She decided to quit her job and launch a career as a technology entrepreneur, launching an app for mothers. "If the assault hadn't happened, I'm not so sure I would have taken that leap. But it happened and, within two years, my app was available on ios. I think society believes women in their late forties are planning for retirement and slowing down, but I'm just getting started on my second act."

For Julie, it was a random event that kicked off a series of changes that ultimately ended up transforming her life. "Ten years ago, when I was in my late forties, I had a car accident," she explains. "That accident made me stop and take a serious look at my life." While she was happy with her life and everything she'd accomplished—"I'd had a business (a salon), I'd owned property, I'd already travelled quite a bit"—she also felt motivated to make some changes. "I ended up reconnecting with, and starting a relationship with, a childhood friend who had adult children of his own," she explains. "We both enjoyed the outdoors, camping, boating and travelling, and so I ended up moving to rural Ontario in my late forties, looking forward to living a simpler life—spending time with his grandchildren and looking forward to his eventual retirement."

Things didn't end up going exactly as planned. Julie and her partner hadn't anticipated that they would join the many grandparents who find themselves raising their grandchildren in the wake of the addiction crisis. They've been raising their six-year-old granddaughter for the past five years. While being thrown into the deep end of parenting at midlife was inevitably a shock, Julie has responded by recalibrating her midlife hopes and dreams. "Something I have learned over the years is that life is an ever-changing path, and even though you can make decisions to guide yourself in a certain direction, you never know what's around the bend." And while what was waiting for her around the bend was something totally unexpected, it's also been something unexpectedly joyous. "Raising our granddaughter has been a joy," she says. "I feel very privileged and honoured to have this opportunity to help raise this child and be a part of our other grandchildren's lives."

Paige also finds herself going through a period of rapid and far-reaching change—in her case, dealing with a series of crises that began to play out during the early months of the pandemic. First the fifty-two-year-old mother of two was laid off from her job, and then things went from bad to worse, with her first-responder husband experiencing a mental health crisis that required in-patient treatment, and with her own painful realization that she had to leave her marriage.

"Had it just been an issue of dealing with the mental health issues, there is no doubt in my mind that I would have been seeing him through this. But there were other things going on and I realized that there was no coming back from some of the things that had happened," she explains. "I'd put a lot on hold and settled for not having my own needs met for a very long time, in an effort to make the marriage work. And I probably would have continued doing that had things not played out the way they did."

The months that followed were all about coming to terms with everything that had changed and trying to figure out what those changes would mean for her and her family from that point on: "It's been a process of supporting my boys through that adjustment and loss, and then having to take a step back and examine what it is that I want from my life. I'm working really hard to model something for my children that I feel is really important: that we can come through this as a family in a way that is about demonstrating respect, kindness and compassion toward one another. I want them to know that you can move through difficult things in a loving way while also having respect for yourself. Because ultimately you have to be able to stand tall and choose what's right, even if it's hard or if it's scary."

And it is really scary, she admitted when we spoke. "I'm standing in a place where I have absolutely no idea what any of this will mean. I have no idea what work will look like, what home will look like, what finances will look like. None of those externals are there for me. They've all fallen away in a year. This is a time for me to grow into something else. I know this is about transformation. I'm still at the beginning of this process—a time when I'm going inward and looking for those places of strength and solace within. And I have that. I know I have the strength to create life anew. Because I've done it many times before."

Claire also takes comfort in that knowledge, the fact that she has a reservoir of inner strength that she can draw upon during times of uncertainty and struggle. "I've always had to be aware of all kinds of different factors, simply because of who I am," the forty-year-old Black woman and mother of two explains. "I've always had to have contingency plans and to battle against challenges that other people might not have."

She's also able to tap into a strong sense of gratitude—the by-product of some important lessons learned in childhood. Before moving to Canada at the age of ten, Claire lived in a small village in Jamaica where daily life was all about meeting some very basic needs. Her family didn't have running water or electricity, so her childhood memories include times spent hanging out in the river while her mother did laundry. And yet she never felt poor. Her needs were being met and she didn't have anything else to compare her experience with.

It wasn't until after she moved to Canada that she realized how different life is for many people in wealthier countries. That has allowed her to feel both grateful for the life she now has and secure in the knowledge that it's actually possible to be happy with a whole lot less. "It's just a very different lens with which to view life," she explains. "A lot of people who come from less are just so much happier in times of stress."

And baked into that recipe for happiness is a new-found ability to tolerate—even celebrate—contradiction. "Lately, I've been looking at the world almost through the process of dialectical thinking to understand that two opposites can exist at the exact same time. I can be exhausted and tired of the pressures of being a Black woman while also grateful to have been born me. I can be up to my neck with the pressures of family life and also completely in love with my kids. I'm happy to be at a point in my life where I am capable of this kind of gratitude and introspection—where I'm finally able to recognize that life is a roller-coaster ride and that's okay."

— CHAPTER 12 —

A Little Help from My Friends

Friendships have always been really important to Alex, but these days she's not feeling like a particularly good friend. Now that she's in her mid-forties, she simply doesn't have the same ability to invest in her friendships as she once did—and that bothers her a lot.

"Friendships have always been so central for me," the psychologist and single parent explains. "I grew up in a family where my parents were pretty neglectful, and so I learned early on that it's my friends who are actually my family. Over the years, I've managed to nurture these super-powerful friendships—friendships that mean the world to me. But when I compare the amount of time and attention I was able to devote to these friendships back when I was younger with what is possible for me right now, there's a major discrepancy. And it's not just me. A lot of my friends are feeling the same way—like they're being pulled in a million different directions and that they don't have the same capacity to invest in their friendships right now. I'm hoping that things will get easier again when my daughter is a little older and doesn't need me as much as she does right now. I really want these friendships to move to the forefront of my life again. But right now it's really tough."

It *can* be really tough to nurture these all-important relationships at a stage of our lives when we're asked to be all things to all people all at once. Something has to give. And too often that something is the very thing we need the most during this messy and confusing life stage: friendships with other women who are muddling through this messiness too.

The magic of midlife friendships

Friendships with other women aren't just important to Jackie, as she journeys through midlife; they pretty much mean everything to her. "I think the biggest thing that I've learned about midlife is that the more you talk to other women, the better you feel," the fifty-year-old writer and speaker explains. "And, sure, you might spend a lot of time complaining to one another about some of the more negative aspects of midlife. Misery loves company, and all that. But there's something to be said for how good it feels to know that you're not alone, whatever it is you might be dealing with. It's so important to not just suffer in silence. You need some kind of support. You shouldn't feel like you have to go through this alone."

And here's something else that's worth noting: it isn't healthy to travel through life alone—not at midlife and not at any other life stage. There's a solid body of research to demonstrate that loneliness can increase your risk of illness and even premature death. In fact, it's as bad for your health as smoking!

And if you're counting on a partner to be your buffer against late-in-life loneliness, you might want to hedge your bets a little by investing in friendships as well. According to a 2019 study published in *Psychology and Aging*, the current generation of older adults is less likely than previous generations of older adults to rely on a romantic partner for social support and more likely to rely on friends.

Of course, you don't have to wait until the future to start reaping the benefits of these all-important friendships. You can start reaping the rewards in the here and now. Lola, a forty-four-year-old writer and single mother, really values the frank and honest conversations she is able to have with a trusted group of friends, conversations that celebrate the joys and acknowledge the struggles of this particular life stage. "Increasingly it's this core group of friends that get me through this. These women know *everything*. They're the women I talk to about the fact that I've been constipated since child number two was born—the fact that nothing's ever working properly downstairs." These conversations help to counter the too-perfect images of midlife that she keeps bumping up against in other areas of her life, whether she's flipping through the pages of a magazine or scrolling through social media. "There's a glossy veneer over everything, but that's not how life actually is. Real life is messy and weird. And maybe if we were able to admit that a little more often, we'd feel better about our lives." That's what these friendships do for her: remind her that she's not the only person finding midlife messy or hard.

Sandra also considers these kinds of soul-nourishing friendships to be the emotional equivalent of a life raft at midlife. "Friends are so essential," the fifty-year-old freelance communications consultant and mother explains. "I am so blessed with friends who have supported me, laughed with me and cried with me. I am so happy to have friends from high school still in my life, and the amazing gift of new friendships with strong, supportive, creative, amazing women. Friendships are golden, and women at midlife need them more than ever."

Paige, fifty-two, has been able to tap into that support on a daily basis, while weathering a series of painful personal storms this past year: the loss of her job, her spouse's mental health crisis, and, more recently, her decision to end her marriage. Lately, she's been thinking a lot about the far-reaching impact of that support and what it means to both give and receive love as a friend. "I hoped that one thing that midlife would bring is strength in relationships, and it has," she explains. "I have an incredible community of women: friends as well as my sister. I'm surrounded by women and connected with women who hold me up when I don't think I can keep going. There hasn't been a day that's gone by since this crisis began that I haven't received a phone call, a text message, an email, a card in the mail, a basket of care products—just so much beauty. It's the first time I've really been on the receiving end of that much love. I think that's the gift of midlife for women: if you have cultivated and nurtured your relationships with other women, you are never alone."

And chances are, your own personal learning and growth over the years have given you the capacity to be a better friend. "I do a lot more listening than I do talking at this point in my life," says Shauna, fifty-three. "I listen to other women, and I support them. I no longer feel like we're in competition with one another. And I'm also just a lot more authentic. I feel like the filters have really come off."

Claire, forty, agrees. "I love and give with fewer strings attached, not because I want something in return but because I'm grateful for what I have."

Midlife loneliness

Midlife has proven to be a much lonelier experience for Sheila than she had imagined it would be. She'd envisioned herself moving through midlife in community. Unfortunately, things haven't played out that way. The fifty-seven-year-old part-time university instructor explains: "When you're in your twenties and maybe even into your thirties, you have this kind of built-in social circle: the friends you make when you're at school or at work. But then your friends start pairing up and having kids and they start pursuing friendships with other people who are on a similar path. I didn't go there. I didn't choose to have kids. I didn't venture down that same path. And because I don't have a relationship with my original family, other than exchanging a couple of emails a year, I've ended up becoming quite isolated. I often think of it as, 'I don't have a family up, and I don't have a family down.' I hadn't anticipated that life would evolve like that—that a couple of significant choices could have such an impact. I had honestly believed that I'd just keep hanging out with my friends as we grew older. But it doesn't end up being like that."

Annie also finds herself craving the consistency and intimacy of some of her earlier friendships. It's not that she doesn't have any friendships—and she certainly has a large number of acquaintances—but something feels different at this stage in her life. The forty-five-year-old mother of two teenagers, who has a mid-level corporate job, explains: "I have one friend that I run with. We go to races a lot together. And she's probably the person that I would consider I'm sort of closest to. And outside of that, I have tons of acquaintances. There are people that are absolutely lovely to go to lunch with, or to have a conversation with, or to touch base with on a particular issue, like parenting. But these aren't the really deep, deep kinds of friendships I remember having when I was younger. That's what seems to be missing for me at this age: the intimate friendships that I remember having back when I was a teenager or in my early twenties." Her gut instinct is telling her that this is a stage-of-life issue. "Everyone is experiencing a time crunch right now. Even if I somehow manage to find time in my schedule, then it becomes a challenge to find time in someone else's schedule, and I'm left feeling like I'm pestering that person all the time. I wish it were less of a challenge."

Angela—a forty-three-year-old doula, yoga instructor and mother of two—also looks forward to having more time for friendships when she's less caught up in the day-to-day demands of parenting. "I have heard from so many people that it's easier to have a social life when your kids are a little bit older. I am really looking forward to that—to investing in friendships that are not as tied to my children. Friendships that I choose for myself as opposed to just being relationships that evolve out of circumstance."

Kelly shares that hope, and she is encouraged by the way things played out for her mother. The forty-one-year-old government professional and mother of three explains: "When I went away to university, my mother suddenly made a new best friend. They ended up being really close and they're still super tight to this day. So that leaves me feeling optimistic that this is maybe just a season—that there will be another season in my life when friendships can become really important again."

Shymol, an engineer who is in her fifties, is grateful to be reaping the harvest from that next season. Now that her kids need her less and she is no longer living within the constraints of a very controlling marriage, she finally has the time, energy and space needed to invest in friendships once again: "Midlife is a wonderful time, and it opens up so many opportunities. The kids are not small, so you can leave them for a few hours without having to worry." Simple things can mean a lot, like "meeting friends over ninety-nine-cent Wendy's Frosties in the summer or getting together to enjoy a walk," she says. "With different friends you share different parts of your life, with each one holding the key to a different chamber of your heart." Midlife, for Shymol, is all about unlocking that precious friendship joy.

Zeroing in on the friendships
that matter most

The challenges posed by the pandemic have given Sheri an opportunity to think deeply about what she actually values in a friendship. "The pandemic has been a really interesting kind of plot twist for me," the forty-four-year-old mother of three who works in government explains. "It's made me think deeply about who I trust in my life, who I feel I can have conversations with about what feels safe and how we can see one another right now, and who I'm willing to Zoom with at nine o'clock at night, after a full day of staring at screens. It's a much smaller list than I previously would have imagined. And it's kind of interesting for me to notice who's on that list—that very short list."

Jackie has been engaged in a similar process of rethinking some of her friendships. "At midlife, friendship is not about numbers. It's about quality," she explains. At this point in her life—she recently celebrated her fiftieth birthday—she finds herself zeroing in on the friendships that matter most. "Back when I was younger, I wouldn't have had the courage to be able to say, 'I don't think I'm going to invest in this friendship anymore.' But now I find it easier to do that. I think midlife has given me that sense of urgency, like, 'I don't have time for that anymore.'"

And, as it turns out, a lot of us don't have time for that anymore—*that* being poor-quality friendships. Becoming a little choosier about who manages to find their way into our friendship circles is a well-documented midlife trend. As psychologists Tara L. Kuther and Kaitlyn Burnell noted in a 2019 article in *Adultspan Journal*, middle-aged adults report investing in fewer friendships than either younger or older adults. This tendency to zero in on the most meaningful relationships is fuelled by the very same factor as Jackie identified: the realization that time is limited.

In order to create room for the friendships that are really fulfilling, sometimes you have to be willing to prune the ones that aren't. For Julia, a forty-seven-year-old freelance musician who is also the mother of two teenagers, that means letting go of relationships with people who no longer mean as much to her as they once did or who never brought anything meaningful to her life. "I find that, at midlife, you distill things. If a twenty-year friendship isn't working for you, you're not going to carry it around for another twenty years, right? At some point, you simply have to decide, 'I'm done with that. That friendship had its moment, but now that moment has passed.'" It's okay to let some relationships go in order to make room for others, she adds. "For me, that means investing in friendships with people who build me up, make me feel good and who are similar to me in terms of values."

Michele is engaged in a similar process of relationship pruning. "As I've gotten older, I've become more conscious of who I spend my time with," the fifty-six-year-old human resources consultant and mother of young adults explains. "I seek out people who help to energize and reinvigorate me, people who are purposeful and joyful and who are interested in having meaningful conversations. I have this one group of friends—a group of women I went to university with—and we have stayed connected over the years. Every summer we get together. We've been doing this since we were in our forties and we've done it every summer since, other than this year, when the pandemic prevented that from happening. When we get together, we sit there and, for three days, we solve all the problems of the world. We talk about ourselves, our lives and our families, and we reflect on all our hopes and dreams for the future. That's the kind of thing I'm looking for—those moments of connection that leave you feeling so good."

Those are the friendships that are definitely worth keeping—or resurrecting again, as the case may be. And that brings to mind a personal story about something that happened to me this past year. While I was researching this book, I had the chance to reconnect in a really powerful way with my very first friend: the friend I made when I was four years old. Marjory and I had stayed in touch in a casual way over the years, but this was the first time we'd sat down (via Zoom!) to truly acknowledge everything that friendship had meant to both of us, back in our growing-up years. This was one of those intense girlhood friendships, a friendship that spanned more than a decade and that laid the groundwork for the girls and women we would become. That friendship is the reason I became a reader and then a writer.

Visiting with my friend allowed me to engage in the best kind of emotional time travel, the kind that sheds light on events that happened in the past—but in a way that also helps to illuminate the present. It's a visit that immediately came to mind when I was reading a recent article by midlife friendship researcher Michelle Piotrowski. Piotrowski noted the impact of long-term friendships—how these friendships allow midlife women "to feel profoundly known and intensely understood over time," and what a gift it is to have a friend who was "a witness" to your growth and personal development, and who is deeply familiar with your history. That's what this conversation with my friend felt like to me: a profound experience of bearing witness and paying tribute to our friendship and shared history.

Jennifer also finds herself appreciating the unique beauty of long-term friendships—and, more specifically, her friendship with her former university roommate Danielle. What the fifty-year-old self-employed mother of two young adults loves most about this friendship is the sense of continuity that it lends to her life. "We might only meet up in person a couple of times a year and talk on the phone a couple of times on top of that, but there's always this sense of a continuing conversation. It's one of the few threads that has continued through my entire life. It's a relationship that is rock solid. It will continue until we die. And it's such an important touchstone for me, knowing that I can call her and just get back to that baseline, no matter what other craziness is going on around me."

Joanna has learned not to take these kinds of precious friendships for granted, after experiencing a searing loss five years ago. "One of my closest friends died very suddenly from a heart attack, basically just walking from his bedroom to his bathroom," the forty-six-year-old accountant and mother of two recalls. The experience of losing this friend really hammered home for Joanna what it means to be at this point in our lives. "People get cancer, people get sick, people are in accidents, and suddenly those people are gone. And along with losing those people, you lose that sense of invincibility. It's a stark reminder of what it means to be at midlife—that you will go before others and others will go before you. And it frames what's important in very significant ways."

Joanna's friend's death didn't just change the way she sees the world. It also changed the way she chooses to *be* in the world. "After his death, I really started to prioritize relationships. I started being more intentional about my friendships, specifically setting aside time to be with my friends. Roughly once a week, I'll make a point of doing something to consciously make memories with friends both new and old. I'm not a shopper. I don't enjoy buying stuff. I like *doing* stuff. And when you share that doing—when you're actively building memories with another person—that really fleshes you out as a human being. It doesn't have to be a big thing or an expensive thing. Sometimes I'll just say, "Do you want to come over and help me pull carrots out of the garden? I'd love to have some company." I try to show up for people in all kinds of ways, including all kinds of fun ways. I am forty-six years old and definitely still appreciate sleepovers!"

"Do life together"

Wendy is a firm believer in the importance of doing life together. In fact, she's adopted it as her tagline. "My job at the church is to get people connected via small groups," the forty-eight-year-old mother of three, who is currently pursuing a master's degree in theological studies, explains. "I'm always saying that to someone: 'Do life together.' And by that I mean find someone with whom you have something in common and find a way to connect. Put yourself out there. That's what it takes to make friends at our age: you have to be willing to be vulnerable and you have to be intentional."

You wouldn't think that people at midlife would need a crash course in making friends, but making friends at midlife can, in fact, be quite different from the way it was when we were younger. We might not be coming into contact with quite as many new people as we once did, and some of the people we do come into contact with might not necessarily be in the market for a brand new friend.

Trying to make new friends can feel like a risky venture, but there's a lot to be gained if you're willing to take that risk, says Melanie, a forty-six-year-old pharmacist and mother of two. "It all comes back to the idea of the village. We don't need to parent on our own, we don't need to go through this midlife journey on our own. We need to have people around us, and that means learning how to make friends at this stage of the game. I now have a very good friend—someone I meet with every two weeks to go for a walk—because the two of us were willing to have that kind of open and honest conversation one day. We talked about how hard it can be to meet people now that our kids are no longer involved and how much each of us wanted to make new friends. And that's how we ended up becoming friends."

Of course, not every woman finds it easy to be that vulnerable. Kelly, for example, has been much more guarded about her friendships in recent years. "I left a lot of friends behind after my son Jeremy was stillborn," the forty-one-year-old government professional and mother of three explains. "That experience made me realize that people aren't always who you thought they were. I lost some of my trust in people. And so building and maintaining really deep friendships is harder. Being vulnerable is harder. I've become a lot more careful."

And just as Kelly is working hard at being more vulnerable, Alana is making a point of being more intentional. She finds herself in a bit of a transitional phase when it comes to her friendships, keeping some relationships and letting other ones go. The forty-three-year-old government relations and policy consultant has been spending a lot of time thinking about which friendships are—and aren't—working for her, and why. "What I'm experiencing in my friendships at midlife reminds me of what happens when you first head off to university," she explains. "You start meeting a whole bunch of new and interesting people but, at the same time, you still have all your existing friends, people you knew in high school and that you're not quite ready to let go of yet. But as the year goes on, you realize that those old friendships don't quite fit anymore. You're in a new and different place in your life. That's kind of how things feel for me right now when it comes to friendships. As I'm progressing through my forties, I'm really digging into my career. That separates me from friends who are emerging from a really intense period of parenting. They're ready to have more fun at the same time as I'm busy working a sixty-hour week."

She's also finding that she has less in common with friends who don't share her passion for social issues, which is leading her to wonder what friendships are going to look like for her from now on. "Do you make a conscious decision to only invest in relationships where you feel like your values are appreciated? Or do you accept that some of the people you hang out with don't care about the same things as you do and are simply interested in living their lives day-to-day? Do you start looking for a new tribe? Or do you accept the fact that you may never again have the same kind of tribe as you had when you were younger? That's kind of where I'm landing at the moment. I'm trying to figure out what relationships I need in my life to feel happy and content and what I want my life to look like a couple of decades from now, given that I'm a solo dweller."

One thing she knows for sure is that she'd like to feel a lot less lonely. That, for her, has been one of the biggest disappointments of this stage of life. "I didn't anticipate midlife having these kinds of stretches of loneliness. I think that's the hardest thing. There are so many times when you just end up doing things on your own. Midlife isn't nearly as community focused as I had imagined it to be. I had a vision of myself being surrounded by other people who you could turn to if you needed something. I'm finding it's a whole lot harder to tap into that support than I had realized. People want to be support-ive, but they're busy. And I'm living on my own. It can take a lot of effort to access that support."

That's also got her thinking about being on the giving–rather than the receiving–end of that kind of relationship, and what kind of family member, friend and community member she'd like to be. "I hope I can continue to be useful and to be of value–to be there for people when they need me. Whether that's leaning in as a daughter, whether that's being a supportive friend for other folks in my life who might need it, or really leaning into my community when it's going through hard times, like it is right now. Those are my hopes and dreams for myself–and what I want for other people too."

— CHAPTER 13 —

Family Matters

It's easy to assume that Elizabeth's life is completely idyllic. After all, she's a visual artist who lives off the grid on an eighty-hectare (two-hundred-acre) parcel of land in rural Ontario. And yet her life is anything but picture-perfect: sandwich generation pressures are an ongoing source of stress for her. She's constantly scrambling to meet the needs of her husband (a teacher), her two children (a preteen and a teen) and her eighty-four-year-old mother, who has a small apartment in their house.

And as for what ends up getting squeezed out of that sandwich? The answer is simple: *herself*.

"Having my parent become more dependent and my children still needy, and doing the majority of the housework, while juggling my career, has left me feeling exhausted and spread thin," the forty-nine-year-old confesses. "I feel like I don't adequately focus on any of these things and especially that my career suffers because, being self-employed, my work time doesn't get prioritized."

When Elizabeth says she's carrying a heavy load, she isn't kidding: "My kids and husband rely on me as a household manager who coordinates appointments, meals, school deadlines and many other basic necessities. Living off the grid, I am also the one who ensures that there is enough wood in the house, that there is gas for the generator, that the septic system has been emptied, that the chickens have been fed. So I am the bearer of this mental load." Her mother also requires an increasing amount of hands-on help with various tasks, but this is help Elizabeth is happy to provide. "My mother enriches our lives and has supported me with words and deeds my whole life. While she struggles with guilt about her inability to help out, she is the one I am happiest to assist because of all the selfless caring she has done for me and others."

While Elizabeth may seem to be carrying an exceptionally heavy load—one that quite literally includes carrying firewood—her experience serves as a great example of how varied our midlife family relationships can be. This is, after all, a time in our lives when those relationships tend to be both abundant and complicated, when our very definition of "family" can be in flux as a result of far-reaching changes rippling through our lives.

Sandwich generation pressures

Utter the words "sandwich generation" anywhere within earshot of Lola and you're guaranteed to elicit a passionate response. The idea that midlife women are the gooey layer that holds that midlife sandwich together isn't just some abstract concept for this forty-four-year-old mother of three. It's a daily fact of life for her and pretty much every other midlife woman she knows. "Every woman I know who is this age is going through the same shit. Sick parents, children who are struggling with mental health issues, problems at the school—there's always something. And we women are expected to be the strong ones, to carry the burden. It's relentless."

And yet it wasn't all that long ago that scholars were busy debating whether, in fact, there even *was* such a thing as a sandwich generation—whether it was common for women to feel "sandwiched" between the competing demands of other generations. Some argued that, by the time elder-care issues show up on the radar for most midlife women, their children have reached an age where they no longer require quite so much hands-on parenting. But while that might have been the case for a brief time in the early 1990s, that's definitely not the case today. As statisticians Melissa Moyser and Amanda Burlock noted in a recent report for Statistics Canada, "Delayed childbearing and transitions to adulthood, as well as population aging . . . increase the likelihood that both children and elderly parents [will] need support from middle-aged workers." And sometimes there are additional generations—a brand new grandchild, a great-aunt—who require hands-on help as well. As a result, that late twentieth-century sandwich has morphed into something a whole lot thicker and messier—more of a club sandwich than a simple sandwich, as human development scholar Karen L. Fingerman likes to put it.

And as for what it feels like to be caught in the middle layer of that sandwich? It's definitely all about feeling squeezed. There are so many competing demands on your time, energies and emotions, says Jennifer, a fifty-year-old mother of two young adults. "Dealing with aging parents with multiple physical health and mental health issues, and who are becoming more and more difficult and less able to show compassion for others, has been a really big challenge. There are many lows on this front. Similarly, watching my kids struggle to find their footing (or regain their footing after a tumultuous adolescence) has also been really difficult for me."

Navigating between cultures and between generations can put an additional squeeze on the generation in the middle. This is the situation that Audrey, a fifty-seven-year-old immigrant person of Asian descent who is also the mother of three young adults, finds herself grappling with on a daily basis. "I feel like I'm straddling two worlds. I'm trying to raise my kids in a particular way—a way that emphasizes both fairness and respect and that is sometimes very different from my own upbringing. This isn't easy for my mother, who may be living here in Canada but who is still very much a product of her culture and generation. And it isn't easy for my kids, who often have a visceral reaction to something she says or does. It ends up being a big burden for me, trying to navigate both worlds and explain things to both generations when no one is really hearing the other side."

The cost of caring

Relationship work—and care work in general—is hard work, but it's meaningful work. The frustration, for many women, is that it's undervalued and often invisible work—and work that women are disproportionately asked to do. A 2020 report published by Oxfam included a couple of truly mind-blowing statistics: women are responsible for three-quarters of unpaid care and two-thirds of paid care work performed globally, and the monetary value of this unpaid care work is "at least $10.8 trillion annually—three times the size of the world's tech industry."

Elizabeth wishes women weren't merely acknowledged for the magnitude and importance of that work (although, frankly, that would be a nice start); she'd also like to see women actually being compensated for it. "Recently, I caught wind of the Wages for Housework feminist campaign of the 1970s. I think that idea [compensating women for their unpaid labour] totally makes sense. Perimenopause has made me more prone to feeling angry about being taken for granted at home, especially as everyone in my house is capable of doing their part but can't be bothered. From my perspective, the most mind-numbing and thankless type of labour involved in child care and elder care is housework: cleaning, laundry and cooking. In an ideal world people would be compensated for this work at home."

And in that ideal world, government policy and funding priorities would acknowledge the structural inequalities that occur when women are required to work for free to an extent that men are not. As Ashton Applewhite points out in her book *This Chair Rocks*, "A society that views caregiving as a private burden rather than a shared necessity disadvantages women, who perform the vast majority of this unpaid or underpaid work. It's unfair, it's exhausting, and it limits women's participation in professional and public life." Which, in turn, has as far-reaching impacts on our finances and our health.

In her book *In Our Prime: How Older Women Are Reinventing the Road Ahead*, Susan J. Douglas makes the case for a fundamental rethinking of the role of government, one that is anchored in the politics of care. She encourages women, who play such an important role in this invisible economy of care, to insist on more and better care-economy investments and supports from government. The kinds of investments that would be life-changing for so many women—and so many midlife women in particular.

Midlife parenting

Parenting requires a lot of investment—emotional, yes, but financial too. And that investment is now continuing well into young adulthood: human development researcher Karen L. Fingerman found that parents across income brackets were typically spending 10 percent of their income on young adult children. In a 2017 article, she noted that this represents a significant shift. While the teen years were the years requiring peak financial investment from parents from the 1970s through the 1990s, since 2000 it's been the early years (prior to the age of six) and the young adult years that have required the greatest cash outlay. How dramatically has the situation changed? Some scholars have reported that over one-third of the financial costs of parenting are now being incurred in the years after children turn eighteen.

The emotional investment has grown too. The relationship between young adult children and their parents has become "more chosen and voluntary in nature," according to Fingerman, but also more emotionally demanding, too, with parents typically having contact with their child at least once a week and with well over half of parents connecting with their child on a daily basis.

By the time they reach their early forties, roughly eighty-six percent of women have become mothers, which means that parenting continues to be a fact of life for the majority of midlife women. But what that actually looks like in terms of the daily lives of individual women can vary tremendously. While some women may have teenagers who are getting ready to leave the nest or young adults who are busy establishing their own lives, others may still be busy chasing around toddlers or scheduling parent-teacher interviews at their child's elementary school. And, of course, some midlife women find themselves caring for children of a variety of different ages and arriving at parenting in many different ways: as a stepparent, a grandparent and so on.

Suzanne, fifty-four, finds herself wearing a couple of those different hats. She's a mother of five and a grandmother of three. At this point in her life, a large part of her work as a parent is finding a way to be a little less caught up in her children's emotional highs and lows. "When I imagined what it would be like to be at this stage of parenting, I envisioned freedom. It never occurred to me how much you still end up worrying about your adult kids. Right now, I'm trying to find a way to detach a little from my children and their choices. I have to keep reminding myself that I've done my best and that now they're off in the world, making their own decisions. I'm my own person and I need to focus on my own successes and failures.

"I'm trying to focus on just loving them, having that—the love—be the bridge between us. I'm trying to find a way to love them as they are, with all their imperfections, so that they can find a way to love me, with all my imperfections."

As Suzanne has discovered, while there are many upsides to the fact that midlife adults and their children tend to be very enmeshed in one another's lives, there can be some significant downsides as well. The emotional toll can be considerable. As midlife development researchers Frank J. Infurna, Denis Gerstorf and Margie E. Lachman noted in a recent article in *American Psychologist*, the impact of having even just one grown child who is struggling can be substantial, fuelling both parental anxiety and guilt.

And the more extreme the struggle, the more extreme that impact can be. Marlene, who describes herself as an Indigenous community activist, single mother and grandmother who is easing into her sixties, has been having an especially tough time. Her daughter's struggle with addiction has forced Marlene to play a much more hands-on role in both supporting her daughter and raising her granddaughter than she had anticipated playing at her age. "My daughter lives with me, in the basement of my house. After being in a state of recovery for about three years, she relapsed recently. And as is often the case with relapse, she fell even harder this time. That's been really difficult for me to deal with as a parent.

"But there is a bright spot, and that bright spot is my granddaughter because, like all grandparents everywhere, I think she's the most amazing thing. I'm raising her half of the time and the other grandparents have her the other half of the time. I love spending time with her, but I hadn't really anticipated being the babysitting grandmother. Before I started providing all this care, I'd started taking painting courses and doing more writing, and now I'm back to making lunches and looking for lost mittens! But here I am. I'm the one who's providing the primary care while her mother takes on the fun kind of aunty role. The unfortunate thing is that our situation is not unusual. I know a lot of [Indigenous] grandmothers who are raising their grandchildren right now. We're losing a generation to the opioid crisis and the meth crisis, in much the same way as we lost earlier generations to the Sixties Scoop and residential schools."

Marlene has discovered that the only way to get through something this hard is by being open and honest with other people about the extent of the challenge she is facing. "At first, I was trying to maintain this brave front, but after kind of breaking down at one point, I realized it would be healthier to talk about what I'm going through, not just for my own sake, but also for the sake of other people who may find themselves dealing with this. I think it's important to show other people that sometimes things aren't okay, that we're not our Facebook selves, that we're real people who have issues and that things like this happen in all sorts of families. We need to be able to talk about what we're going through so that we can get the help we need and be a source of strength to one another."

Community is a thread that has run through Marlene's entire life, regardless of where she's been living. "My band membership is with a community I've never had the opportunity to visit—Lax Kw'alaams on the West Coast—but I grew up in a small community in Manitoba where everyone had to help each other," she explains. "It was a community with a one-room school, a place where the parents ended up fundraising to get the snowplow to plow the road, a pioneer setting where community meant everything." And, once again, community means everything to her—the friends who listen, understand and offer support to her and her family.

Not all happy families

Sometimes when things fall apart, they fall apart in a major way.

In Jude's case, that falling apart involved a devastating rupture in their relationship with their child—an experience that came dangerously close to breaking them.

"When my son was twelve, he went to his dad's as scheduled and never returned," the post-secondary administrator, who is in their early forties, explains: "He'd been splitting his time fifty-fifty between his two homes for ten years." It was a moment that changed everything. "Legally, his father and I have joint custody, but my son does not want to live with me or even see me. At the time of this writing, it has been nearly three years since he lived with me and it has been sixteen months since I saw him, albeit very briefly. He will occasionally correspond by text but is fairly nonresponsive and continually refuses to see me, even during the pandemic, when I just asked him to come to his bedroom window so I could see his face."

While this kind of experience would be shocking for anyone, it was particularly devastating for someone who had invested so much of themselves in parenting. "I spent 2018 grieving this huge loss. Who was I if I wasn't mothering? What life did I have when I wasn't in the thick of parenting a child with a long list of diagnoses? I had no idea who I was outside of being a mother. I say that 2018 brought me to my knees. I really don't know how I managed to make it through those first twelve months alive. At one point, I ended up taking myself to the emergency room because of overwhelming thoughts of suicide."

Since that time, Jude, who describes themselves as non-binary agender, has focused on their own health and mental health, and on creating a new life for themselves—a life that meshes with the painful reality that they continue to be estranged from their son. "At the beginning of 2019, I started a job in an entirely different sector and have been selective about what I share. I try to avoid mentioning that I have a son because, the moment I mention I have a teenager, it's assumed that I'm navigating the school system and monitoring Instagram accounts and so on, when, in actuality, I don't know what he looks like and how he's navigating adolescence as a trans teen or what shoe size he's wearing or how long his hair is. We used to talk about the books we were reading. I used to nag him about cleaning his room. We used to fight over his refusal to eat anything that wasn't beige. But now I have to navigate several layers of school bureaucracy and to reference the Children's Law Reform Act, just to receive a copy of his report card.

"While I no longer dread coming home after work, knowing that there will be an angry teenager waiting for me, the cost of that is immeasurable. I hope that no one else ever has to deal with a situation like this, because there is no support around grief and loss when it comes to an estranged, alienated child. I thought I had many more years of having my child in my home and navigating school advocacy and health systems for his medical transition. And then, all of a sudden, I was no longer parenting, and I didn't know what to do with my time."

It's painful to read about family estrangement, let alone live it, but Jude wants other people to know that this can happen, because family estrangement is something that isn't talked about nearly enough.

Georgia, the fifty-seven-year-old mother of two young adults, also wants to break that silence, which is why she's chosen to speak about one of the most painful experiences of her life: the end of her relationship with her mother. More specifically, she wants people to understand that long-standing problems in families don't magically disappear, just because everyone is growing older. In fact, they can go from bad to worse to, in her case, completely irreparable.

People who haven't lived through this kind of relationship rupture can find it difficult to understand how something like this could happen, she says. "There can be a lot of judgment. People say things like, 'How could someone stop talking to their mother? They must be an awful person.' I need people to understand that it's not that simple. My mom suffered from mental health issues and psychotic delusions for her entire life. And what made a bad situation even worse was the fact that I had no family support in dealing with her. Everyone else kept pretending that she was just fine, but she *wasn't* just fine. I also need people to understand that this isn't the kind of decision you take lightly. When someone gets to the point where they need to cut off contact with a family member, it's not just a matter of, 'Oh, I don't get along with that person.' It's more about there being no infrastructure left within that family. The fact that there's nothing left to work with." And, even after her mother's death, that continues to be the case. "When my mom died, my sister never called me. I found out through a relative. They either never had a funeral or they didn't invite me."

A few key realizations have helped Georgia to make peace with the situation. "I remind myself that she was ill, that none of this was my fault, that there is nothing I could have done to make the situation better, that I kept her in my life for as long as I could—and that there's no point in having any regrets."

Midlife couple relationships

Midlife can be a high-pressure time for couple relationships—a time when marital satisfaction levels have a tendency to hit rock bottom, before climbing steadily higher again during the post-parental years of marriage (assuming, of course, that the partners haven't decided to exit the relationship entirely by that point).

It's a phenomenon that Jodi, a fifty-year-old marketing executive and mother of two, has been observing in her own life. "I think the love and marriage piece is kind of taking a back seat right now," she admits. "I give a lot to my kids, I put a lot into my career, and that means my marriage sometimes ends up getting squeezed out. It's as much my fault as anyone's. I know I could do better. And yet this is how it is. I think it will get easier over time. When I think about the things that stress out a marriage, it's disagreements about the kids, money pressures, time pressures—things that will probably be less of an issue as the kids grow older. I feel pretty confident that, once we get through this stage, things will be really good again."

Joanna has also been thinking about the future—about all the exciting plans she has for herself, and how she hopes her husband will find a way to fit into those plans. That's required some tough conversations because, as it turns out, the two of them originally had very different visions of what the next couple of decades might look like. While he's getting ready to gear down, the forty-six-year-old accountant and mother of two is getting ready to gear up. "I remember him saying, 'What if I want to retire?' And I said, 'That's great! You can volunteer with some of the projects I'll be doing.' And then he said something that made my heart sink: 'Isn't this enough for you?'"—meaning their marriage, their family, their life. And for Joanna, the answer to that question was no. *No, it wasn't enough.* "It's not that I don't love all the things about our family and our life. I do.

But I also think there needs to be more. The idea that my life is going to be exactly like this forever feels really crushing to me. It leaves me feeling really trapped. I need to be able to look to the future in a way that says, 'What else can I do while I'm here?' We ended up having an honest conversation about our lives—one in which I was able to say, 'I'd love to have you come along, but this is going to be my time.'"

For some women, shifting their focus to the future means recognizing that they want something different and better for themselves—something more than may be possible in the context of their current relationship.

"Middle age for me started out in a place of really questioning life," says Shay, a forty-eight-year-old single mother of two and grandparent who is also the executive director of a non-profit. "I started asking myself if I was happy with the life I had. I'd been married almost twenty years at that point, and yet I kept thinking, 'I feel like there's more to life. I don't know that the husband, couple of kids, decent job and house is everything that I want.'"

Shay started re-evaluating her life and rethinking her options after reflecting on her mother's early death. "My mother died four days after she turned fifty," she explains. "She had been diagnosed with cancer at forty-nine. It looked like she might make it, but she didn't. The time from diagnosis to death was eight months." This got Shay thinking about how quickly a life can pass by—and what it would feel like to reach the end of your life with a lot of your own personal hopes and dreams still unfulfilled, because it was pretty clear that this was how things had played out for her mom. "I remember having conversations with my mom, back when I was in my late twenties—conversations in which I'd asked her, 'Are you happy with your life?' And she'd say, 'I would like to have done so much more, but I got pregnant; and, at that time, in the early '70s, when that happened, you got married and you raised your kids.'" And then Shay's mother would talk about how she was biding her time until the day arrived when her youngest child was finished college, because that was the day when she was going to start to live her life. "The year she was diagnosed with cancer, my brother actually had just graduated from college. He graduated that May, she was diagnosed that July, and then she died the following March. And so, entering middle age, I kept thinking about the fact that my mother gave her whole life to raising kids, taking care of us, and she never got to do the things that she wanted to do."

Recognizing all the things that her mother had missed out on made Shay realize that she needed to start being much more intentional about the choices she was making. And that meant rethinking whether she wanted to continue to stay married to an admittedly really great guy, because it was becoming increasingly clear that the marriage was no longer working for either of them. "I remembering thinking, 'Do we really want to be those people who realize, when they reach their sixties or seventies, that they should have split up a long time ago? And do we really want to let the relationship deteriorate to a point where we don't even like each other anymore?' Because we all know people like that—those older people who should have admitted to themselves years ago, 'It was a good run, but now we're done.'" For Shay, it was about making a conscious decision to end things on a positive note: "To leave honouring what we had for almost twenty years; to leave while we were still able to say, 'I like you.' And six years later, my ex-husband continues to be one of my best friends. He's one of the few people in the world that I trust."

Midlife has also been a time of increased self-awareness for Lola, a forty-four-year-old writer and mother of three who recently made the decision to end her second marriage. "I think that something I have realized (and it took me two kicks at the can to figure this out) is that marriage is not for me and maybe relationships in general—long-term relationships with men—aren't for me either. I feel like I've given up way too much of my life to looking after way too many people. And as for the emotional labour thing? I simply don't have it in me to do that ever again."

When Lola looks around her, she sees a lot of other women drawing this same kind of line in the relationship sand. "I know a lot of other women my age who are suddenly realizing that they really don't want to live with a man anymore. And I know a lot of single women who never got with a man in the first place—women who always seemed to be a whole lot happier than I was."

And while ending a marriage inevitably involves a lot of emotional upheaval, Lola is finding her way to that happier place. "I was brought up to believe that you need a man to look after you, and that you're nothing if you don't have a man. Those messages were ingrained in me from a very early age. And now I feel like I've reached a point in my life where I'm able to recognize that I don't need anyone to look after me—I'm perfectly capable of doing that—and that it's possible to get my emotional needs met in all kinds of other ways, including my deep friendships with other women and the affection of my children. Ending my marriage has created more room for these relationships because I'm no longer trying to cram in all the stuff I was trying to cram in before. I feel like I'm finally getting that need for a man—that need to be validated by a relationship—out of my system."

Lola isn't the only woman to weigh the pros and cons of marriage and decide that the "pros" column is sorely lacking. A study led by psychologist Johanna Drewelies concluded that marriage has become a decidedly less appealing proposition for women over time. Not only have women become less dependent on marriage as a source of financial security and social support, but they're less likely to feel happy about shouldering a double load, attending to everything that needs to be done both at home and at work. Many women are responding to that unappealing proposition by either taking a pass on marriage entirely or choosing to walk away later on. And when someone makes the decision to end a marriage, that someone is overwhelmingly a woman—and it has been for some time. As sociologists Sarah Milton and Kaveri Qureshi noted in a recent article, "By the 1990s, nearly three quarters of divorces were initiated by women."

Jennifer Lawrence, a forty-eight-year-old divorce coach who describes herself as "happily twice-divorced," spends a lot of time in the company of women whose marriages are ending. She's found that the majority of her clients are happier post-divorce than they were while they were still married, and she's come across some data that supports what she's been seeing with her clients: "A recent study showed that three-quarters of women do not regret their divorces, even if they weren't the ones who initiated them. Women tend to be happier post-divorce, in part because for the first time in years, they are acknowledging what they want and meeting their own needs. They're embracing their independence."

That pretty much describes where Alex finds herself four years after the sudden and unexpected end of her marriage: embracing her new-found freedom. That's not to say that the process of getting there was easy. The forty-five-year-old single parent had to trudge through a lot of emotional muck. "It doesn't matter how shitty your entire marriage was," she says. "When it finally comes to an end, it's still a shock, because it's finally done." So first she had to deal with the shock and then she had to start recalibrating her dreams—completely reimagining what her future would look like. "The year I turned forty-one, my marriage started to dissolve. I hadn't expected that to happen. I'd thought that I was happily married. I had two kids and we lived in the suburbs. We had a good life, and I was a stay-at-home mom. Then everything that I'd known to be true for the previous twenty years of my life started to dissolve, and within two years everything was gone."

What helped her to get through this really painful time was the support of other women who'd been through the same experience, and who were willing to be real about both the struggle and the opportunity. Yes, it's hard to let go of what was, but it can be exciting to imagine what could be. And while her new life includes a partner—a part-time partner who doesn't live with her—her priority at this stage of her life is taking full advantage of her new-found freedom. "It's very freeing to be 100 percent comfortable going to sleep, just me at night, and waking up, just me. I like having a partner, but that relationship no longer defines or limits me. I love being with someone who values my independence. It just feels so free."

Of course, what feels liberating to one woman can feel like a loss to another. While Suzanne didn't regret the end of her marriage, she isn't loving being single. "When I separated from my husband, I honestly assumed I would meet somebody within the next couple of years and that within five years I'd probably be remarried to somebody great. But that didn't happen. That person never showed up," she explains. And while the fifty-four-year-old mother, grandmother and birth worker's life is rich in relationships, she often finds herself feeling really lonely. "I have always had a really rich friend life, family life and community life. Always. And that's still the same now. I'm really blessed in that way. But, at the same time, I'm super lonely. I really miss having a partner."

Alana hadn't necessarily anticipated that she'd continue to remain single after a ten-year relationship ended a decade ago, but she's okay with the way things played out. "I think I did envision, at this point in life, being partnered. But that hasn't been my path and I don't know if it will be at any point." While she's not in any big hurry to start dating again, at the same time, she hasn't slammed the door on that possibility. The experience of one family member has taught her that you can never be totally sure what the future might have in store for you. "My solo-dwelling, independent great aunt got married for the first time at age sixty-eight, to the man she fell in love with at eighteen!" But as for those friends who keep telling her that she needs to start dating again, she's quick to point out, "I'm cool. I have a puppy."

Rebecca has chosen to take herself off the dating market altogether. The fifty-two-year-old social worker, who has been divorced for the past thirteen-and-a-half years, has realized that she no longer has the emotional energy needed to sustain a romantic relationship. After her marriage ended, she had tried dating for a while, only to realize that the needs of her kids and the demands of her job didn't leave her with a whole lot left to give. "I didn't think it was fair to put myself out there under false pretenses—to try to pretend that I was going to be the best girlfriend, wife or whatever in the world. Because I'm not. I have other priorities. I give a lot to my kids and my friends. And when it comes to the emotional part of relationships, I like to tell people, 'I gave at the office.' I'm a mental health and addiction social worker. I only have so much to give."

— CHAPTER 14 —

Differently Political

Midlife is a time in our lives for standing up for ourselves and for one another, for daring to acknowledge all the things that should be better and looking for opportunities to make a difference—in our families, our communities, our world.

"Midlife women are a force to be reckoned with," says Lisa, a forty-four-year-old anti-violence educator, activist and researcher. "So much of what has been accomplished in social justice movements over the years has been accomplished by strong and resilient women, mostly at midlife, saying, 'That's enough. Things need to change.'"

This chapter is about leaning into our power as audacious midlife women. It's about recognizing how much power we actually have when we come together to work for change, and how much richer and more meaningful our lives become as a result of those efforts—the joy that comes from being part of something bigger than ourselves and looking for the unique opportunities in our own lives to do whatever we can to nudge the needle of progress in the right direction.

It's time . . .

There's something about this particular life stage that seems to fuel a desire for change.

It could be the result of our time perspective suddenly flipping. As developmental psychologist Alexandra M. Freund explained in a recent article in *American Psychologist*, when we're younger, we tend to focus on how long we've lived, but once we hit midlife, we start thinking more about how much time we have left. That growing sense that time is limited could definitely help to ramp up the sense of urgency that so many of us feel. As Darcey Steinke notes in her midlife memoir *Flash Count Diary: Menopause and the Vindication of Natural Life*, "For the first time, I feel like I have a time stamp, an expiration date."

It could be because we have a growing sense of the bigger picture. We're able to connect the dots between what we've experienced in the past, what we're living through right now, and what we'd like to see happen from this point forward. As Mary Catherine Bateson noted in her book *Composing a Further Life: The Age of Active Wisdom*, "As you think further into the future, you see more and more inter-connections, and your concerns extend more widely as well, like a swath of light extending through a partly opened door into darkness."

And it could be because midlife women have a tendency to function as a bridge between generations—the generation that both connects and supports the generations that came before and those that will follow. "Midlife is, and has always been, about relation-ships—about the roles we play in the community and in the family, the sacrifices we make, the experience we bring to bear," writes Susan P. Mattern in her book *The Slow Moon Climbs: The Science, History, and Meaning of Menopause*. "We become non-reproductive so that we can do other things . . . Menopause is necessary. Humans have menopause because we need it. The contributions of post-reproductive women have brought us this far and will lead us into whatever future we have."

And if all of this sounds pretty political, that's because it is.

The mere act of living, and of being a woman, is political.

Trish Hennessy would love to see more midlife women conceiving of themselves as political beings—connecting the dots between the personal and the political. The director of Think Upstream, a non-profit think-tank that focuses on identifying policy solutions for fostering a healthier society, believes that midlife women have the potential to be a powerful force for change.

A crucial first step, according to Hennessy, is allowing yourself to be audacious enough to imagine a better future for yourself and others. "When I look back on my hopes and aspirations when I was younger, I can't help but marvel at my audacity. Here's a kid coming from rural Saskatchewan, growing up in a large farming family, where we basically lived off the land, and somehow wiping the muck off of my boots and moving to the city to pursue a university education—the first in my immediate family. I hope I'm as audacious heading into the final chapter of my life.

"And, speaking more broadly, audacity is what I hope for the world moving forward, because the challenges we face, collectively, are immense. COVID-19 has exacerbated already intolerable levels of income inequality. Precarious work is on the rise. Our communities will continue to be challenged by climate emergencies. Women, especially racialized and immigrant women, will be disproportionately impacted by these challenges. We all have a role to play to hold our governments to account, to ensure governments invest in policy decisions that can address these challenges—the greatest gift this generation of women could give future generations. My greatest hope is that we organize, advocate, educate and take comfort that with the gift of age comes a different kind of power. We need to champion audacity, and each other."

"I thought things would be so
much better by now"

Lately I've been trying to figure out when it was that we first started using the term "dumpster fire" to describe a really bad year—and when we collectively decided to stop using that term, because it had pretty much lost all meaning. At what point did we finally acknowledge that we were living in what amounted to a non-stop dumpster fire?

While I haven't managed to pinpoint the dates exactly, it seems that we latched on to the term a year or two before Donald Trump was elected—and then, once that unthinkable thing had happened, there simply wasn't any reason to retire the term. And then, of course, we found ourselves heading into a pandemic. All of which is to say that the past few years have been rough—really, really rough—for anyone who happens to be a caring, thinking person.

If you happen to be around the same age as I am (which I'm assuming you are, given that you're reading this book), you grew up hearing a lot about the inevitable forward march of progress—something that doesn't feel nearly as inevitable or forward-moving anymore. In fact, in many ways, it feels like progress has done a complete about-face—that much of the progress that has been made over the course of our lifetimes is actively being dismantled or even erased. It's been both disorienting and devastating.

The months following the election of Donald Trump were a particularly low point for many women.

For Deb, a fifty-one-year-old political communicator for a union, Trump's rise to power felt like a deeply personal kind of loss—something very different from anything she'd ever experienced before. "I've been political for most of my life, and I've been political in all kinds of different ways, so I'm used to dealing with election losses and campaign setbacks," she explains. "But when Hillary lost—and I wasn't even a huge fan—I was utterly devastated. It was one thing for her to lose, but for her to lose to him of all people. It took me months to get over that. In fact, I'm not even sure I'm completely over it, even now. I think part of my psyche was permanently damaged by that experience."

Shelly, a fifty-eight-year-old who works for a small non-profit organization, found herself reeling from the results of the election combined with the relentless barrage of deliberately cruel policy decisions that followed. "It was terrifying to watch so much ground being lost so quickly, so much of the work that had been done over a matter of decades being erased," she recalls.

And that was just the beginning, notes Kristine, a fifty-year-old arts worker: "The election of Donald Trump gave the world licence to be trash."

The hardest thing for Carolyn, a forty-nine-year-old mother who works in health care, has been realizing, in the years since Trump's election, just how much work is left to be done if she's going to witness anything resembling social justice in her lifetime. "I thought life would get better as I got older. I felt like I would have to fight less. But that hasn't proven to be the case at all," she says.

Rather than having the luxury of coasting through this chapter in her life, she's been ramping up her activist work—and doing what she can to bring the next generation on board. "I took my daughter to the Women's March in DC. It proved to be a very pivotal moment in my life, realizing how close we were to losing everything and seeing women older than me carrying signs that read, 'We were here in the '70s and we're still here fighting this bullshit.' That made me realize that this fight is likely to continue for the rest of my life—that I'm going to be that woman in her nineties, sitting there with a sign that says, 'I'm still wearing my pussy hat. We're still here!'"

And if the Donald Trump years kicked off a process of soul-searching for a lot of midlife women, the pandemic amplified and intensified that process. For many, it became a multi-layered experience of pause: the pandemic pause layered on top of the self-reflective pause that is so characteristic of midlife. It was no longer possible to go on with our lives as usual because ordinary life had ground to a halt—and suddenly we were being forced to rethink everything.

It was a liminal moment, a rupturing of routine, an opportunity to pause long enough to consider what was and wasn't working. As Jenny Odell explains in her brilliant and thought-provoking book *How to Do Nothing: Resisting the Attention Economy* (which, incidentally, was written back in pre-pandemic times), sometimes that kind of pause can serve as a launching pad for change: "Most people have, or have known someone who has, gone through some period of 'removal' that fundamentally changed their attitude to the world they returned to. Sometimes that's occasioned by something terrible, like illness or loss, and sometimes it's voluntary, but regardless, that pause in time is often the only thing that can precipitate change on a certain scale."

That's certainly Paige's hope—that we'll act on some of the important learning that has been happening over the course of the pandemic. For the fifty-two-year-old, who has experienced a lot of far-reaching upheaval in her own life during this time, that means learning to tolerate uncertainty and to accept the fact that there are often no simple or easy answers. "I really hope that we can choose to live with questions instead of racing for answers, so that there's space for the right answers to rise. I like living with questions," she explains.

Alana, a forty-three-year-old government relations and policy consultant, also wants things to be different. And not just different– better. *So much better.* In fact, while she's painting me a picture of what better could look like, she has to pause for a moment to regain control of her emotions. "We've got big challenges and big fights ahead of us in this world and we need to do better," she says. We need to be more creative about how we solve these problems, whether it's inequity or climate change or poverty or the impact of technology or war. I just want things to be better. I just want *us* to be better."

The good news is that there are a whole lot of us who want things to be better–and a whole bunch of different ways to work for change. Instead of feeling crushed by all the things that need to be fixed, we can feel heartened by the number of hands that are willing to do the work, and the number of different ways there are to contribute to that effort.

We can build on the efforts of all the caring people who came before–and we can blaze a trail for the changemakers who will follow in our footsteps, long after we're gone. And we can tap into our own unique opportunities to contribute during the time that we're here.

The future is older and it's female

Here's something fascinating that our youth-centric media has a tendency to overlook: the future is older, and it's female. As May Chazan notes in the introduction to *Unsettling Activisms: Critical Interventions on Aging, Gender, and Social Change* (a book she edited with Melissa Baldwin and Patricia Evans), "Over the next 35 years, the global population over the age of 60 is expected to triple, so that by 2050, for the first time in history, there will be more people over 60 than under 15. Life expectancy is higher for women than it is for men, with populations over 60 estimated to include two to five times as many women as men."

And not only are there going to be a lot of us, but we're going to continue be a force to be reckoned with throughout midlife and beyond. "Evidence suggests that women remain politically engaged longer than previously recognized—many are actively working for social change well past the age of sixty-five," Chazan writes.

What's interesting is that many midlife women don't consider themselves to be political when, in fact, they're quietly (or not so quietly) working for change in all kinds of different ways and in all kinds of different areas of their lives. While there may be times in their lives when women are engaged in few outwardly visible acts of activism, this doesn't necessarily mean that they've disengaged. It might simply mean that they've chosen to be "differently political" for now.

Because here's the thing: there are all kinds of different ways to be political. Being political doesn't have to mean grabbing a picket sign and heading out the door to a protest. It can also mean finding ways to live your life in a way that reflects your values—engaging in the "small, daily acts of resistance [that have] the potential to create broader change," as May Chazan, Melissa Baldwin and Jesse Whattam, who coined the term "differently political," point out in their essay for Unsettling Activisms.

For Jean, being "differently political" has meant shifting her focus from being political in a very public way to "bringing activism home." The fifty-three-year-old writer, academic and mother of three explains: "To other people, it might have looked like I hit the pause button on all my activist work but, in reality, I had brought activism home. We adopted three kids from high-trauma backgrounds and, for a while, while we focused on meeting their needs, there simply wasn't energy or time or money or anything left to give to the rest of the world. And while I know that that's not widely perceived as activism, it was for me. And while I continued to care deeply about other issues—in particular, I became acutely aware of the way our culture fails to support the parentless, the homeless, the traumatized—I recognized my limits. I only had the power to help the ones who lived in my house."

Politics have also become a whole lot more personal for Alex in recent years. While there's so much more she'd like to be doing on the activist front, the psychologist and single parent who is in her mid-forties also recognizes that she has limits, and that, for now, her seven-year-old daughter needs to be the priority. "When I start feeling really weighed down by how little activist work I'm able to take on right now, I remind myself of how much energy I'm putting into my parenting: 'At least I'm home loving my child. At least she's going to get a decent start.' That's something my parents weren't able to do for me, and I know the price I had to pay for that. So, for now I'm really focusing my efforts on reversing that pattern—at least as much as I can."

Louise finds it helpful to remind herself that the deep capacity for caring that she's developed during the really hands-on years of parenting is a resource that she will be able to share with her community over time. "I hope to shift the mothering and caregiving I've been giving for the last two decades to my community and society," the forty-seven-year-old mother and writer explains. "I feel I have flourished in this role, and I don't have any intention of turning it off. As my kids need me less (though really, do they ever need you less?) I want to channel my energy into caring for a wider population. I feel we already do a fair bit as a family, but with fewer domestic and child-rearing demands, I look forward to doing more."

Christine takes comfort in the fact that the job of fixing the world doesn't rest entirely on her shoulders and that it's okay to step in and out of various volunteer roles as time, energy and life circumstances allow. In other words, she doesn't have to be doing all the things, all the time. "I don't need to fix everything," the forty-eight-year-old writer and mother explains. "There are lots of people working for change."

And if you think about it, that's our superpower as midlife women: the power of numbers. There are a lot of us, and we've accumulated a lot of life experience. Even wild elephants have figured out that it's the older matriarchs you want to turn to in times of trouble. They're the ones who have lived long enough to know where to find food and water in times of drought. And they've learned how to spot patterns, so they're able to anticipate potential problems. That makes them an invaluable resource.

Human society would do well to take a similar approach, notes Julia, a forty-seven-year-old freelance musician and mother. "By the time women reach midlife, we've been keeping society going for a long time. Instead of just ignoring us, maybe listen to us a bit—because we actually have a lot to offer."

Making change together

Veronica is a fierce believer in the power of community. In fact, she pretty much lives and breathes community. "Creating and sustaining communities is what I do," the forty-six-year-old Latina educator and mother explains. "I do that for a job. I do that in my spare time in the community. I am a community organizer in my neighbourhood. I try to ignite and cultivate conversations around our lives—what we need from each other, what we need from our elected officials. And I've also been a reproductive justice activist for many years. Everything I do is connected to either sustaining or creating a community with a feminist lens, with an eye toward making the world a more just and beautiful place."

That's not to say that working for change is easy. In fact, at times it can be really hard. The pace of progress can be frustratingly slow—and then, of course, there are all the roadblocks and setbacks you inevitably encounter. This is why being part of a community of others who share your vision for a better world is so important. What makes it possible to keep going is the fact that you're doing this work with others. "I have a lot of friends who turn to me when they're feeling really frustrated—when they feel like they've lost their enthusiasm for the work," says Veronica, noting that, when this happens, she tries to encourage those friends to focus less on each person's individual efforts and more on what they are able to achieve as a community of women working together. "Let's say we're talking about smashing the patriarchy. I encourage them to think of the patriarchy as this huge, huge slab of rock—and to imagine each of us with our own little chisels chipping away at that rock. If we just keep picking up whatever chisel we have and chipping away as much as we can, eventually we'll get there—we'll manage to smash that rock."

What will ultimately cause that rock to collapse into a heap of rubble will not be the actions of a single person but rather the cumulative efforts of a large group of people relentlessly chipping away over a prolonged period of time. As feminist gerontologist Martha Holstein points out in her book *Women in Late Life: Critical Perspectives on Gender and Age*, "Individual acts of resistance and agency will not alone, in the long run, change the system. Resistance, to be comprehensive, needs to systematically involve many people in some organized way." We need a whole lot of people wielding their chisels.

And it all starts with women comparing notes about the realities of their lives—recognizing that it's not just you or me who wants things to be better than they are. It's pretty much all of us. Imagine what could happen if, instead of focusing on the kinds of changes we can make on our own, we actually dared to consider the kinds of changes we can make together. That's how social movements are born!

Trish Hennessy is definitely on that same wavelength. Lately, she's been thinking a lot about the small-group conversations that fuelled the activism of second-wave feminism. "When I went back to university in my late-twenties and all through my thirties, I kept reading about the feminist movement in the 1960s and '70s, how women would meet, educate, agitate. We're a long way from that but there's much to learn from that era of organizing."

Lisa, a forty-seven-year-old activist, academic and mother, agrees: "Maybe what we need is a good old-fashioned consciousness-raising circle."

And as for what we might talk about in that circle and what kinds of issues we might want to organize around? Let's start with the structural factors that conspire to make life challenging for women of all ages, and that can really start to snowball by midlife—the rigid gender norms that are at the root of so much of our suffering and the fact that patriarchy casts such a wide shadow (and supports so many other interconnected systems of oppression).

Audrey, a fifty-seven-year-old political staffer and mother, knows exactly what she'd be talking about if she were hosting that kind of discussion over a pot of coffee in her living room: "Everything from the traditional gender roles that we're forced to take on, whether we want to or not, to being taken for granted in terms of everything we contribute to society." Even though the inequality she has experienced as an immigrant person of colour living in Canada has been less blatant than what she experienced growing up in a country where women were routinely treated as second-class citizens (and where racial tensions complicated issues of inequality even further), she resents the fact that things aren't better than they are, especially given how much rhetoric there is about everyone in Canada being equal. "Life is very unfair to women. There are so many missed opportunities and unfair expectations, and I think, for a lot of women, that breeds a lot of resentment. Sometimes I like to joke (and I'm not really joking) about how, in my next life, I'd like to come back as a man. I say that because I feel like they have it pretty good."

Audrey would also like to see more people flexing their empathy muscles—expanding their capacity for caring. "I get frustrated with friends and neighbours whose approach to life is really insular—who don't care about an issue unless it has a direct impact on their families or people just like them. Their lives are set up in a way that they have the luxury of not having to think about a lot of other things. In other words, they have a lot of privilege."

For Sheri, a forty-four-year-old mother of three who works in government, responding to that privilege means challenging herself to continue to learn and grow as a person, and to look for ways to translate that learning into action. "You really have to seek out other perspectives or you're not going to change," she explains. "And that change is going to feel uncomfortable. Now that my kids are a little bit older and I have a little bit of capacity, I'm back to wanting to be uncomfortable, in the sense of experiencing that kind of change. It's like when you work out. When you're sore, you know you've really done something that's going to change your body. And that's where I'm at with activism. It needs to hurt a little bit in order to feel like it's changing me." She's working her empathy muscles, in other words. And she's also committed to continuing to support the efforts of other women—Black and Indigenous women—who are leading movements aimed at dismantling white supremacy. "I don't feel like I have the right perspective to be out in front of anything. I don't *want* to be out in front of anything. It's more about being a listener and a follower."

Comparing notes with other women—a diverse group of other women—is a powerful way to learn about interlocked systems of oppression. As progressive think-tank director Trish Hennessy explains, advantage (or disadvantage) accumulates over time, and yet "we don't grow up talking about these intersecting factors and how they trail you throughout life." Instead, we look at life through a very individual lens, thinking that it's all about personal choices. Or we feel overwhelmed by the day-to-day realities of life and at the mercy of our circumstances. What we so often miss are the broader, more systemic factors that are at play, including the daily political decisions from all levels of government.

Connecting these dots is super important because even the most seemingly mundane policy decision can have far-reaching impacts on our lives, Hennessy explains. Take, for example, "the municipal government that refuses to invest in sidewalk snow clearing because of the cost, rendering moms with strollers and young kids as well as people with disabilities invisible" (and, by the way, people with disabilities are more likely to be women than men). That supposedly straightforward budget-cutting exercise has a very gendered impact. As Hennessy points out, "Sidewalk snow clearing is a feminist issue."

And that's just a single policy.

Zeroing in on your own opportunities to make change

When you stop to consider all the things that are in serious need of fixing, it can all start to feel pretty overwhelming. That's why it's so important to make an effort to zero in on your own unique opportunities to make things better, in ways both big and small. As Ezra Bayda points out in *Aging for Beginners* (a book he wrote with Elizabeth Hamilton), "The more we can truly understand that we don't have endless time, the more we can connect with what really matters to us—which allows us to prioritize more clearly how we really want to spend our time and energy."

For Suzanne, it's a matter of considering where she's most likely to have an impact. "As I've gotten older, I've become a whole lot clearer about what I can and can't change," the fifty-four-year-old explains. "Back when I was in my twenties, I was very idealistic. I thought that I could change the world. But now I realize that there are only so many hours in the day, that I only have so much energy, and that I need to spend that energy wisely. I've also come to understand that no single person can save the world. There needs to be a groundswell in order for that to happen. I'm only one person and I have a limited sphere of control—a limited ability to make change. And so I choose to focus my energies on that: making the change that I can. That's been a really big shift for me."

For Kel, an activist and mother in her mid-fifties, it means being increasingly selective about what she is—and isn't—willing to take on at any given time. "When I was younger, I used to always say yes to exciting projects. I now know that learning to say no is a necessary journey. At this stage in my life, I am fortunate to be able to pick and choose projects that I believe will have the most impact, and that is where I focus my attention."

And for Deb it means knowing when she needs to take a break from her activist work entirely. "I've gotten a bit better about taking a step back, just engaging in whatever way I need to, whether it be with a hobby or mindless television or my dogs," the fifty-one-year-old political communicator explains. "Knowing more about myself and how deeply I feel things—and how deeply I am affected by what other people are feeling—I've learned the importance of giving myself the time and space I need to recover so that I can come back and do it again."

Sometimes the most radical thing you can do is to take a break yourself and to look for an opportunity to pass the baton to others. Rather than burning yourself out, you're choosing to safeguard the precious resource that is you and to build up capacity in others at the same time. This has been a key piece of the learning that Joanna has been doing at midlife: shifting her emphasis from "What can I do?" to "What can we do together?" "These days, it's more about empowering the people around me—using my skills to support other people, and sustaining all the relationships needed to make things happen," the forty-six-year-old, who is involved in numerous community projects, explains.

Sharing the responsibility and the workload also relieves some of the pressure to achieve a particular goal during your lifetime—something that may not even be possible, given the magnitude of whatever it is you're working toward. "This is one of the benefits of being part of a community," says Claire, a forty-year-old non-profit founder whose advocacy work focuses on maternal mental health. "If I reach a point where I'm no longer able to do the work, I know that there are other people who are ready to pick up wherever I leave off because there are already so many people out there doing similar work. It's not a matter of me needing to accomplish something myself. It's more a matter of doing what I can before it's time to hand off the baton to the next person. It's not about any individual person reaching the finish line. It's about all of us getting there together as a result of our collective work over the years."

Lori also has a strong sense of being part of something bigger than herself—a movement of people who are working for the kind of change that can't necessarily be achieved in a lifetime. "If we're all pursuing the same kinds of goals, then the beginnings and the ends get woven together," the fifty-four-year-old organizer, activist and campaigner says. This way of looking at things has helped Lori to work through some of her grief about the deaths of some of her fellow activists. "It was so difficult to lose these women—women my age—and the best way I know to honour them is by carrying on with their work."

As I'm speaking to Lori, a powerful image pops into my head: a beautiful striped scarf that represents the work of a whole bunch of different knitters, each contributing their own kind and colour of yarn. Where one knitter's work ends, the next knitter's work begins, with the scarf growing longer and more beautiful over time.

The long view of progress

If there's one thing that Veronica, forty-six, has learned during her many decades as a community builder, it's the importance of taking a long view of progress—of recognizing that making meaningful gains takes time. "I am a student of organizations. I spend a lot of time thinking about how systems work—how hard it is to overthrow an entire system. This is why I'm an incrementalist. I understand that the radical overthrowing of *anything* rarely happens overnight. It takes a while. And so we need to have a long game."

What encourages her to stick with that long game are the generational signs of progress that she's witnessed through her work as an educator and activist. "People who were on the front lines [of the women's movement] in the '70s and the '80s—and then those of us who took up the mantle of the '90s—have had children or we've worked with young people in educational spaces. We've worked hard at raising up a generation of more enlightened, empathetic, justice-minded humans. Each generation builds on itself—and we're just starting to see the fruits of all that earlier labour."

Shay, a forty-eight-year-old Black woman who is deeply immersed in anti-racism work through her job as the executive director of a non-profit, envisions herself planting seeds for a future harvest—a harvest that will happen long after she's gone. "My strategy is to accept that racism is not going to be resolved in my lifetime, that the work we're doing right now to start to move toward something better is a matter of planting seeds," she explains.

"I'm a grandparent. I have a four-year-old grandson. I don't think things are going to change in my lifetime. They're probably not going to change in my kids' lifetimes. Maybe they will change in my grandkid's lifetime." Because it's not just a matter of planting those seeds; it's also a matter of planting those seeds in the right kind of soil—soil that is actually able to support and sustain that crop. At this point, we don't have the right kind of soil. We won't have the right kind of soil until the broader culture is willing to stop pretending that everything is fine and face some really uncomfortable truths, she explains.

At this point, Shay switches analogies, telling me a story about a home reno project that almost did her in because she wasn't willing to acknowledge some deep underlying problems. "Years ago, when I was with my husband, we bought a house that was built in the 1880s. A Victorian-style house. The kind of house that, if you were handy, which we were not, you could really do a lot to fix it up. So anyway, most of the rooms had wallpaper, but it wasn't just any kind of wallpaper. It was that really nasty wallpaper: horsehair plaster. You really have to have particular skills to take the wallpaper off. Otherwise, you just ended up messing up the walls. So at one point I was so frustrated with the whole process that I decided to just start painting over the wallpaper. And here's the reason that I'm telling you this story: I feel like that's what we tend to do about our deep societal issues, especially around race. It's 'We're just going to paint over that ugly wallpaper and not remove anything.' And yet the real change won't happen until a plurality of white-bodied people are willing to face the truth."

They also have to be willing to act upon that truth, she adds. "I think a lot of white people get stuck feeling guilty for being white. And to that I say, 'Look, you didn't have a hand in deciding what race you got to be. You are what you are.' And am I saying that you need to feel bad about something that happened four hundred years ago? No, but you do have to recognize it. And you also can't just get stuck on, 'Well, I know I have white privilege.' Okay, that's great. So how are you using that privilege?"

Like Shay, Celina Caesar-Chavannes had hoped to witness more change being made on the racial justice front over the course of her lifetime. The forty-six-year-old former parliamentary secretary to Canadian Prime Minister Justin Trudeau, who documented the racism she encountered as a Black woman in politics in her explosive memoir *Can You Hear Me Now? How I Found My Voice and Learned to Live with Passion and Purpose*, remembers attending a high-profile racial justice protest back when she was a teenager. A couple of decades later, she found herself marching again—in this case, to protest the murder of George Floyd. "Did I think that we would be further along at this point? Absolutely. Because we've been here before. I often talk about the fact that I attended the protest in Toronto in '92 when Rodney King was beaten in the United States, how we were marching in the streets saying, 'No justice, no peace.' And yet here I am again, in 2020, bringing my kids to a protest to speak out against the very same kind of brutality against Black bodies." This makes her wonder what the future will hold—whether there will be any meaningful progress on issues of racial justice or whether she'll end up being "the woke grandma who is taking her grandkids to protests thirty years from now."

So how do you hold on to hope when progress feels incremental, or when you're witnessing the loss of a lot of hard-won gains?

For Lori, it's a matter of reminding herself that other generations have also been forced to deal with devastating setbacks, and yet they chose to keep working for change regardless. "If I look at history, I can see that I'm not the first person to feel devastated by a particular result, nor will I be the last. History teaches us that we can find a way to bounce back—and that the work we are doing does make a difference."

For Joanna, a forty-six-year-old accountant and mother of two who is actively involved in numerous community projects, coping with disappointments and setbacks means becoming more strategic in her activist work. "These days, I'm all about the order of operations—what needs to happen in what order to make things happen. I think that's the wisdom piece for me. I used to just want to jump in. But now I'll stop to consider how I can be most effective. It's one of the benefits of being at this point in our lives—having the benefit of so much practical experience. You remember all the holes you've fallen in."

For Shauna, a fifty-six-year-old social entrepreneur who recently entered the race to become the mayor of a major city, it's about looking for ways to build resilience in herself and others over time. "I think we are in for a very long emergency," she explains. "This is a tough time we're in. And I'm not just talking about the pandemic. Climate change is going to continue to manifest itself in many different ways. So how do we create resilience over the long term? How do we create the kinds of conditions in which all of us can thrive? For me, that means moving away from ideas of scarcity and toward ideas of collaboration, community and belonging."

That brings to mind something author and chaplain Kate Braestrup said in a 2016 interview on the radio show *On Being*: "The question isn't whether we're going to have to do hard, awful things, because we are. We all are. The question is whether we have to do them alone."

And this is what I choose to believe: we don't have to do those hard things on our own. We can journey into that unknown future in the company of others who share our vision of a better world. And even if we don't manage to fix all the things that are in desperate need of fixing (a pretty safe bet, I think), our lives will be richer and more meaningful, simply by virtue of the fact that we tried.

And that, for me, is the biggest reason I'm drawn to various types of volunteer and activist work: because of the joy and meaning it adds to my life. Yes, there are times of tremendous frustration. Yes, I get my heart broken on a regular basis. But am I ready to give it up? Not on your life.

It's worth doing the work because the work is worth doing, regardless of the immediate outcome, or whether, in fact, I even manage to see significant progress in my lifetime. As Margaret Urban Walker notes in her book *Mother Time: Women, Aging, and Ethics*, when women look back on their lives, their most treasured memories are inevitably of times when they had a small role to play in something bigger: "a relationship, a family, a political movement, a partnership, an enterprise, an institution, a creative process, a ritual event."

I also like the person I become—and the people I get to know— while I'm doing that work. "Anger isn't just a blaze burning structures to the ground; it also casts a glow, generates heat, and brings bodies into communion," writes essayist Leslie Jamison. I crave community because I crave that kind of communion—relationships forged in moments of shared outrage *and* shared joy. Because community is both life-enriching and life-sustaining and because, at this point in my life, relationships mean everything to me. And if I'm lucky enough to do my part to help nudge the needle of progress in the right direction, well, what more can a person ask from a life?

Jackie is asking herself these same kinds of big questions as she works at finding that sweet spot between feeling too responsible for solving all the world's problems and feeling that nothing you could possibly do will ever really matter at all. Not that standing on the sidelines is even an option for her, given that she's the mother of a Black child. "I don't have any delusions that I'm going to single-handedly change the world," the fifty-year-old writer and mother explains. "But I really want to spend the remaining years that I have, however long that may be, feeling like I am doing something positive, that I'm doing something that will allow my daughter to say, 'At least my mom tried. She didn't just turn her back on the world's problems.'"

Midlife Reimagined

We can choose to rethink the very idea of midlife: to treat it as a unique and important life stage in its own right, as opposed to merely an inconsequential stopover in the journey between youth and old age.

We can celebrate the many ways midlife contributes to our growing sense of self-awareness and self-knowledge. For many of us, that means reconnecting with cherished elements of our younger selves. As Darcey Steinke puts it so powerfully in her book *Flash Count Diary: Menopause and the Vindication of Natural Life*, "One of the clear gains of menopause has been a resurgence of my fierce little-girl self. My passion, taken up for a while with the domestic, now lasers out into the wider world. My sense of injustice is sharper and I want to resist." (I think Darcey and I may be leading parallel lives.)

We can recognize it as a time of continued growth and flourishing. Philosopher Hanne Laceulle makes the case for telling stories about midlife that are anchored in "narratives of becoming" that acknowledge both the losses and the gains that tend to accumulate by midlife, and that are real about what is (and isn't) within our power to change. Midlife is neither magical nor miserable. We are neither powerless nor all-powerful. The truth is (as always) somewhere in the messy middle.

We can treat it as an opportunity to invest in relationships. Instead of buying into our culture's fierce insistence on independence—and of living with the fear of becoming a "burden" as we grow older—we can choose instead to celebrate our glorious interdependence as humans. As Mary Catherine Bateson notes in her book *Composing a Further Life: The Age of Active Wisdom*, "The reality of all life is interdependence. We need to compose our lives in such a way that we both give and receive, learning to do both with grace, seeing both as parts of a single pattern rather than as antithetical alternatives." We can choose to view our inevitable reliance on other humans as a blessing, not a burden. As Ashton Applewhite points out in her book *This Chair Rocks: A Manifesto Against Ageism*, "Autonomy requires collaborators. Establishing and nurturing those relationships makes a lot more sense than fetishizing self-reliance." Midlife is a great time to start conspiring with potential later-in-life collaborators and forging friendships with women of different generations, and planning to journey through the remainder of our lives "with one arm stretched out to those who are older than ourselves, and the other reaching back to those who will follow in our footsteps," in the words of narrative psychologist Molly Andrews.

We can recognize the radical potential of midlife—and by that I mean the opportunity to make change. Yes, this is a stage when we are increasingly treated as invisible, and we can recognize that invisibility for what it is: a kind of superpower. "My friends and I have started to see our ability to fly under the radar as a real opportunity," says Martha, a fifty-nine-year-old communications professional. "People make assumptions when they see the grey hair. One day they're going to wake up and realize that we're actually ninja feminists, that we've infiltrated everything and that nothing is ever going to be the same again!" And in terms of how we might want to use those feminist ninja superpowers for good? I like Trish Hennessy's idea about leaning into our power as "audacious" women—women who refuse to settle for a badly broken status quo and who aren't afraid to raise their voices and insist on better. And I'm constantly inspired by political scientist Shirin M. Rai's call for "a shared good life"—a life that's deeply rooted in caring for one another. But above all, I want us to continue to work for the kinds of change we've been waiting for our entire lives, and to love one another through the messy process of figuring out how we make that change together.

And finally we can treat midlife as an opportunity to honour the uniqueness of our own journeys—the unique combination of life circumstances that brought us to this place and made us who we are. "There is not one path through midlife but rather a complex variety of passages," write Nancy Mandell, Susannah Wilson and Ann Duffy in their book *Connection, Compromise, and Control: Canadian Women Discuss Midlife.* "Because their lives [do] not unfold in the predictable, linear fashion they were raised to anticipate they would, midlife women find themselves with many opportunities for creative reconstruction . . . The paths [through midlife] are not clearly articulated; women must find their own ways."

The good news?

We don't have to make that journey on our own.

We can journey together.

We can continue to share our lives and our stories.

Afterword

This may be the end of the book, but I'm hoping it will mark the beginning of a broader conversation about what it actually means to be a woman at midlife. I'm hoping that this book has inspired you to reflect on the joys, challenges, meaning and potential of this one-of-a-kind life stage and that you'll look for opportunities to share some of that thinking with other women. And in an effort to nudge that process along, I thought I'd share the list of questions that I drew upon in my interviews with the women who spoke with me for this book. They're the kind of questions that you might want to sit with for a while, journal about (assuming you're the journalling type) or discuss with a trusted group of women you know and care about. Bottom line? I honestly don't want this book to end. I hope you're feeling the same way. This list of questions is my attempt to keep the conversation going.

- What does society get wrong and right about what it's actually like to be a woman at midlife?
- What were your expectations of midlife? How have those expectations measured up to the reality? What would younger you find most surprising, most frustrating or most exciting about the way your life has turned out and/or the person you've become?
- What have been the high points and the low points in your own personal journey through midlife? What lessons have you

learned or insights have you gained from these experiences? What strengths have you developed along the way?
- What does the view from midlife look like for you? Do you find yourself looking backward or forward? In what ways are you able to connect the dots between past, present and future? In what ways are you able to spot evidence of both continuity and change?
- What are your hopes and dreams for yourself, your family, your friends, your community and our world—and what role do you see yourself playing in attempting to realize those hopes and dreams?

Acknowledgements

It would be impossible to write a book like this without the behind-the-scenes support of a huge number of people.

I am incredibly grateful to the women who agreed to be interviewed for this book and who gave me the gift of trusting me with their stories: Veronica Arreola, Kim Ashbourne, Sara Bingham, Lisa Black-Meddings, Janet Bolton, Amy Brown, Lola Augustine Brown, Andrea J. Buchanan, Celina Caesar-Chavannes, Sarah Campbell, Kelly Carmichael, Shymol Chambachan, Danielle Christopher, Lisa Clarke, Lara Cooley, Angela Crocker, Wanda Deschamps, Deborah Duffy, Nana aba Duncan, Marlene Elder, Melanie Everets-Rodrigues, Paige Stirling Fox, Angie Gallop, Fawn Geddes, Stephanie George, Jackie Gillard, Michele Girash, Louise Gleeson, Sara Gold, Alexandra Gousse, Shelley Divnich Haggert, Sheri Hebdon, Christine Hennebury, Andrea Henry, Joanne Ilaqua, Sandra Ingram, Kat Inokai, Shelly Ives-Sargent, Angela Jackson, Adrienne Jaroslawski, Junia R. Joplin, Cathy Kerr, Christine Klassen, Jane Kristoffy, Lisa Lachance, Julie LaRocca, Jodi Lastman, Alana Lavoie, Jude Lee, Samantha Leeson-McCoy, Suzanne Lim, Lisa MacColl, Danielle Macfarland, Kristine Maitland, Leigh Medeiros, Karyn Methven, Laura Earl-Middleton, Lily May Miller, Leigh Mitchell, Audrey Moey, Jennifer Moore, Kim Moran, Jenna Morton, Lorrie Murphy, Martha Muzychka, Ketha Newman, Rebecca Norlock, Jackie Osmond Patrick, Sarah Pell, Elsa Perez, Angela Petry, Emily Popek, Lucy Porter, Valerie Quann, Shauna Rae, Sharon

Reid, Kelly Ross, Tricia Ross, Rosanna Ruppert, Alana Salsberg, Wendy Saulesleja, Julia Seager-Scott, Shaun Sellers, Erika Shaker, Michele Sparling, Helen Hirsh Spence, Shay Stewart-Bouley, Lori Strauss, Shari MacDonald Strong, Shauna Sylvester, Penny Tantakis, Alexandria Thom, Katrina Urquhart, Eileen Velthuis, Robin Elise Weiss, Kendra Wilde, Sheila Wilmot, Jill Wood, Heather Wright, Jacki Yovanoff, Claire Zlobin and everyone else who chose to share their stories with me anonymously.

I also owe a sincere thank you to the various subject matter experts who were so generous with their time and expertise: Ariel Dalfen (psychiatrist); Jo-Anne Gottfriedson (an Indigenous Elder who is a member of the Tk'emlúps te Secwėpemc people in the Interior of British Columbia); Trish Hennessy (director of Think Upstream); Shaunacy King (menopause doula); Jennifer Lawrence (divorce coach); Christine Luckasavitch (Indigenous author, scholar and cultural consultant); Lisa Petsinis (life and career coach); Sara Smeaton (midlife coach); and Tamara Soles (psychologist and parenting coach).

I truly appreciate the two brilliant and hard-working members of the technical review panel, who put almost as much heart and soul into this book as I did: anti-violence educator, activist and researcher Lisa Clarke and Indigenous author, scholar and cultural consultant Christine Luckasavitch. Thank you for your wise and encouraging feedback.

I am lucky to have friends who both shared my excitement about this book project and who understood when I did my usual book writing disappearing act. (The final stretch of book writing always seems to require me to enter the book world equivalent of the witness protection program.) Thank you for the ongoing gift of your friendship, Lori Bamber, Christine Hennebury and Cathy Kerr, and for literally being my very first friend, Marjory Phillips. And thank you to my activist friends, Michele Girash and Kelly Carmichael, for sharing my faith in the possibility of a better world and for your fierce determination to do the work needed to take us there.

I also need to thank all the people who played a role in helping this book find a home and to make its way out into the world: Hilary McMahon of Westwood Creative Artists (the kindest and most supportive literary agent *ever*) and the super enthusiastic members of my new book publishing family (who seem to be just as excited about working with me as I am about working with them): Anna Comfort O'Keeffe, for her willingness to get behind the book I ended up writing (which was very different from the book I had initially proposed); Caroline Skelton, for offering so much detailed and helpful feedback and encouragement at every stage of the editing process (and in a way that made me feel like I was hanging out with a friend); Merrie-Ellen Wilcox, for being both a brilliant and detail-minded copyeditor and a genuinely kind and helpful human being; Luke Inglis, for all the behind-the-scenes editorial heavy lifting; and Corina Eberle, for being a powerhouse of a publicist and one of the hardest-working and best-organized people I've ever met.

And speaking of family, I need to wrap up this list of acknowledgements with a totally inadequate message of thank you to my family, who continue to be my greatest supporters and champions. Thank you to my husband (Neil), my children (Julie, Scott, Erik and Ian), my sisters (Janet, Lorna and Sandra), my dad and my entire extended family for putting up with me as I switched into author-zombie mode once again. A special shoutout to Neil for spontaneously (and apparently non-ironically) declaring, "I love being married to an author!" at just the right moment—when I was in the very thick of book writing. It seems kind of fitting that we first fell in love at a library, given how much our lives have been centred on books—both the books I keep writing *and* the books I keep buying! (Yes, I know there is limited bookshelf space in our tiny-yet-perfect lakeside home.) I look forward to continuing to write more chapters in the ongoing love story that is us (and maybe another book or two, too).

Notes for Readers Who Want to Know More

Instead of overwhelming you with an exhaustive—to say nothing of *exhausting*—list of every book, article and other resource I consulted while I was researching this book, I've zeroed in on the best of the best: the ones that are actually worth tracking down. Here are the reference materials that proved to be most helpful to me while I was researching each chapter—along with a few quick side conversations, just to keep you reading!

Chapter 1: Hello, Midlife?

Want to get up to speed on the current thinking about *when* midlife happens and *what it's for*? I found myself drawing upon these two articles time and time again. I hope they'll be just as helpful to you too: "Midlife in the 2020s: Opportunities and Challenges" by Frank J. Infurna, Denis Gerstorf and Margie E. Lachman (*American Psychologist*, May-June 2020) and "Mind the Gap in the Middle: A Call to Study Midlife" by Margie E. Lachman (*Research in Human Development*, August 27, 2015).

You may be only a few pages into the book, but you've no doubt already figured out there's a lot of work to be done to ensure that all women are adequately represented in midlife research. For more on intersectionality (a term coined by legal scholar Kimberlé Crenshaw to describe intersecting modes of oppression) and midlife experience, see *The Seven Necessary Sins for Women and Girls* by Mona Eltahawy (2019), *Women in Late Life: Critical Perspectives on Gender and Age* by Martha Holstein (2015) and *This Chair Rocks: A Manifesto Against Ageism* by Ashton Applewhite (2015).

Reading Eltahawy's book encouraged me to seek out the works of other authors who share her commitment to justice and liberation, and who had something unique to add to the midlife conversation. Authors who fundamentally contributed to my thinking while I was writing this book include the following: feminist scholars and researchers May Chazan, Melissa Baldwin and Patricia Evans, whose book *Unsettling Activisms: Critical Interventions on Aging, Gender, and Social Change* (2018) shines a spotlight on how women and non-binary people engage in acts of resistance, resilience and resurgence at various times in their lives and, in particular, at midlife and beyond; narrative psychologist Molly Andrews, whose book *Narrative Imagination and Everyday Life* (2014) makes the case for telling ourselves new and better stories about midlife and, in particular, stories that emphasize "becoming"—our journey of growing into ourselves; disability justice activist, poet and scholar Eli Clare, who boldly challenges life-limiting and ableist thinking about what it means to live with a disability or a chronic illness in his book *Brilliant Imperfection: Grappling with Cure* (2017); journalist Nora Loreto, who makes the case for a stronger and much more intersectional feminism in her book *Take Back the Fight: Organizing Feminism for the Digital Age* (2020); sociologist Jessie Daniels, whose brilliant new book *Nice White Ladies: The Truth about White Supremacy, Our Role in It, and How We Can Help Dismantle It* (2021) explains the role that well-meaning "nice white ladies" like me intentionally or unintentionally play in upholding multiple systems of oppression; and essayist Darcey Steinke—author of *Flash Count Diary: Menopause and the Vindication of Natural Life* (2019)—and historian Susan P. Mattern—author of *The*

Slow Moon Climbs: The Science, History, and Meaning of Menopause (2019)—whose books on menopause caused me to rethink everything I thought I knew about this particular rite of passage.

Chapter 2: Midlife Expectations

A lot of the midlife worries discussed in this chapter had something to do with money. It's hardly surprising, given that women find themselves on much shakier ground financially than men, especially as they grow older. For more on the financial realities of midlife (and how the fact that women continue to take the lead on caregiving work factors into that decidedly unequal equation), see "Born to Retire: The Foreshortened Life Course" by David Ekerdt (*The Gerontologist*, February 2004); "Self-Empowerment in Later Life as a Response to Ageism" by Paul Irving (*Generations: Journal of the American Society on Aging*, Spring 2015); "A Call to Action: Where to from Here?" by Martha B. Holstein (*Generations: Journal of the American Society on Aging*, Winter 2017-2018); "Economic Inequality in Later Life" by Karen D. Lincoln (*Generations: Journal of the American Society on Aging*, Summer 2018); and "Historical Change in Midlife Health, Well-Being, and Despair: Cross-Cultural and Socioeconomic Comparisons" by Frank J. Infurna, Omar Staben, Margie E. Lachman and Denis Gerstorf (*American Psychologist*, September 2021).

Chapter 3: The Messy Middle

Once I started to read about the ageism that's baked into the two predominant midlife narratives—narratives of decline and so-called "successful aging"—I started to spot these narratives everywhere. The books and articles that really helped me to understand why these narratives are so ubiquitous and so problematic were *Agewise: Fighting the New Ageism in America* by Margaret Morganroth Gullette (2011); *Out of Time: The Pleasures and Perils of Ageing* by Lynne Segal (2013); *In Our Prime: The Invention of Middle Age* by Patricia Cohen (2012); "Revisiting Happiness and Well-Being in Later Life from Interdisciplinary Age-Studies Perspectives" by Ieva Stončikaitė (*Behavioral Sciences*, September 3, 2019); "Valuing Old Age Without Leveraging Ableism" by Clara W. Berridge and Marty Martinson (*Generations: Journal of the American Society on Aging*, Winter 2017-2018); "Disrupting Aging" by Jo Ann Jenkins (*Generations: Journal of the American Society on Aging*, Spring 2015); and "On Being an Old Woman in Contemporary Society" by Martha B. Holstein (*Generations: Journal of the American Society on Aging*, Winter 2017-2018).

Of course, we don't have to settle for those two terrible narratives. We can imagine new and better midlife narratives into being. The book that got me really excited about the ways we could do this was *Narrative Imagination and Everyday Life* by Molly Andrews (2013), a really brilliant and inspiring book. And if you're in the mood for some truly wild reimagining, you might also want to treat yourself to a copy of *Braiding Sweetgrass: Indigenous Wisdom, Scientific Knowledge, and the Teachings of Plants* by Robin Wall Kimmerer (2013). Kimmerer's book isn't about aging per se, but the way it emphasizes interdependency and interconnectedness resonated with me deeply, so I really want you to know about this book too. If you'd like to read more about the impact of intersectional narratives, you'll want to read "The Challenge of Intersectionality" by Toni Calasanti and Sadie Giles (*Generations: Journal of the American Society on Aging*, Winter 2017-2018) for theory, and *Age Ain't Nothing but a Number: Black Women Explore Midlife*, edited by Carleen Brice (2003), for some real-life stories.

Chapter 4: Happily Stressed

You've no doubt heard about the so-called U-curve of happiness—the theory that happiness dips at midlife. What you might not know is that there's actually a long-running and quite heated debate about whether this so-called curve actually stands up to academic scrutiny. If you'd like to learn more about the controversy, the following two articles are both informative and entertaining: "The U Shape of Happiness Across the Life Course: Expanding the Discussion" by Nancy L. Galambos, Harvey J. Krahn, Matthew D. Johnson and Margie E. Lachman (*Perspectives on Psychological Science*, July 2020) and "Midlife as a Pivotal Period in the Life Course: Balancing Growth and Decline at the Crossroads of Youth and Old Age" by Margie E. Lachman, Salom Teshale and Stefan Agrigoroaei (*International Journal of Behavioral Development*, January 1, 2015). Then, once you're finished getting up to speed on all that, you might want to round out your knowledge of all things midlife happiness by reading *Encore Adulthood: Boomers on the Edge of Risk, Renewal, and Purpose* by Phyllis Moen (2016), a guide to finding something at least remotely resembling happiness at midlife.

Curious about the origins of the myth of the midlife crisis? *Midlife Crisis: The Feminist Origins of a Chauvinist Cliché* by Susanne Schmidt (2020) is an exhaustive and scholarly book that will have you rolling your eyes anytime you hear the words "midlife crisis" from now on. For a less detailed but more readable take, pick up a copy of *In Our Prime: The Invention of Middle Age* by Patricia Cohen (2012) instead.

For more about stress at midlife (which is, of course, an all-too-real thing), see "Midlife in the 2020s: Opportunities and Challenges" by Frank J. Infurna, Denis Gerstorf and Margie E. Lachman (*American Psychologist*, May–June 2020); "Expecting Stress:

Americans and the 'Midlife Crisis'" by Elaine Wethington (*Motivation and Emotion*, June 2000); "A Life Span Developmental Perspective on Psychosocial Development in Midlife" by Tara L. Kuther and Kaitlyn Burnell (*Adultspan Journal*, April 2019); and "Happily Stressed: The Complexity of Well-Being in Midlife" by Jeffrey Jensen Arnett (*Journal of Adult Development*, December 2018).

Chapter 5: The View from Midlife

I am fascinated by the thinking part of midlife: why midlife is a period of such intense self-reflection and what this means in terms of our own potential for learning and growth. I read a huge number of books and articles related to this theme. These are the ones that I find myself turning to over and over again: *Composing a Further Life: The Age of Active Wisdom* by Mary Catherine Bateson (2010); *Awakening at Midlife: A Guide to Reviving Your Spirit, Recreating Your Life, and Returning to Your Truest Self* by Kathleen A. Brehony (1997); *Breaking Free: Women of Spirit at Midlife and Beyond* by Marilyn Sewell (2004); *Mother Time: Women, Aging, and Ethics*, edited by Margaret Urban Walker (1999); *The Third Chapter: Passion, Risk, and Adventure in the 25 Years After 50* by Sara Lawrence-Lightfoot (2009); *Narrative Imagination and Everyday Life* by Molly Andrews (2013); *Connection, Compromise, and Control: Canadian Women Discuss Midlife* by Nancy Mandell, Susannah Wilson and Ann Duffy (2006); *Women Rowing North: Navigating Life's Currents and Flourishing as We Age* by Mary Pipher (2019); "Storied Worlds: Acquiring a Narrative Perspective on Aging, Identity, and Everyday Life" by William Randall, from the book *Narrative Gerontology: Theory, Research, and Practice*, edited by Gary Irwin-Kenyon, Brian de Vries and Phillip G. Clark (2001); and "The Life Narrative at Midlife" by Dan P. McAdams (*New Directions for Child and Adolescent Development*, Fall 2014).

Sharon Wray's comment about midlife being a time of life where "past, present, and future intersect" comes from her article "Women Making Sense of Midlife: Ethnic and Cultural Diversity" (*Journal of Aging Studies*, January 2007).

My thinking in this chapter was also inspired by a comment James Baldwin once made about the "baffling geography" of midlife (in "God's Country," which was published in the *New York Review of Books* on March 23, 1967). And it was inspired by the article that pointed me to Baldwin's article in the first place: "Imagining the 'Baffling Geography' of Age" by Molly Andrews (*Journal of Aging Studies*, December 2018).

Chapter 6: Self-Acceptance: The Midlife Edition

Most of the material in this chapter was inspired by my conversations with the women I interviewed for this book, but I also learned a lot from *Connection, Compromise, and Control: Canadian Women Discuss Midlife* by Nancy Mandell, Susannah Wilson and Ann Duffy (2006).

Chapter 7: The Truth about Menopause

If you're interested in the physical health aspects of menopause, I highly recommend the following books (and Heather Corinna's book in particular): *What Fresh Hell Is This? Perimenopause, Menopause, Other Indignities, and You* by Heather Corinna (2021); *The Menopause Manifesto: Own Your Health with Facts and Feminism* by Jen Gunter (2021); *Mastering Menopause: Women's Voices on Taking Charge of the Change* by Deborah M. Merrill (2019); and *Our Bodies, Ourselves: Menopause* by the Boston Women's Health Book Collective (2006).

If you're more interested in the socio-cultural aspects of meno-pause, then the books and articles you might want to track down are *Flash Count Diary: Menopause and the Vindication of Natural Life* by Darcey Steinke (2019); *The Slow Moon Climbs: The Science, History, and Meaning of Menopause* by Susan P. Mattern (2019); *In Our Prime: The Invention of Middle Age* by Patricia Cohen (2012); "Women Making Sense of Midlife: Ethnic and Cultural Diversity" by Sharon Wray (*Journal of Aging Studies*, January 2007); and "Multiple 'Old Ages': The Influence of Social Context on Women's Aging Anxiety" by Anne E. Barrett and Erica L. Toothman (*The Journals of Gerontology: Series B*, November 2018).

For more about the incidence and impact of various types of menopausal symptoms, you might find the following articles help-ful: "The Challenges of Midlife Women: Themes from the Seattle Midlife Women's Health Study" by Annette Joan Thomas, Ellen Sullivan Mitchell and Nancy Fugate Woods (*Women's Midlife Health*, June 15, 2018); "The Midlife Women's Health Study—A Study Protocol of a Longitudinal Prospective Study on Predictors of Menopausal Hot Flashes" by Ayelet Ziv-Gal et al. (*Women's Midlife Health*, August 17, 2017); "Work Outcomes in Midlife Women: The Impact of Menopause, Work Stress and Working Environment" by Claire Hardy, Eleanor Thorne, Amanda Griffiths and Myra S. Hunter (*Women's Midlife Health*, April 9, 2018); "Self-Compassion Weakens the Association Between Hot Flushes and Night Sweats and Daily Life Functioning and Depression" by Lydia Brown et al. (*Maturitas*, August 2014); "It Is Not Just Menopause: Symptom Clustering in the Study of Women's Health Across the Nation" by Siobán D. Harlow et al. (*Women's Midlife Health*, July 27, 2017); and "Women's Midlife Health: Why the Midlife Matters" by Siobán D. Harlow and Carol A. Derby (*Women's Midlife Health*, August 11, 2015).

Some of the other materials I consulted while researching or actually referenced in this chapter include *The Middlepause: On Life After Youth* by Marina Benjamin (2016); "Are You There, God? It's Me, Menopause" by Jen Gunter (*Glamour*, October 19, 2020); the "Rethinking Menopause" episode of the CBC Radio show *Ideas* (September 5, 2019), which included interviews with both Susan P. Mattern and Darcey Steinke; the Society of Obstetricians and Gynaecologists of Canada tip sheet "What Is Menopause?" (which I accessed in 2021); Rock My Menopause (a UK menopause information website and information campaign created by the Primary Care Women's Health Forum); "See Fewer People. Take Fewer Showers" by Maria Cramer (*New York Times*, May 6, 2021); and the "Perimenopause" comedy sketch from *Baroness von Sketch Show* (September 30, 2019).

Chapter 8: Midlife Mental Health

For more about the emotional roller-coaster ride of midlife, see *What Fresh Hell Is This? Perimenopause, Menopause, Other Indignities, and You* by Heather Corinna (2021).

Chapter 9: Your Body at Midlife

For more about the realities of living with what feminist gerontologist Martha Holstein likes to call "an attention-demanding body," I recommend the following two resources: *Women in Late Life: Critical Perspectives on Gender and Age* by Martha Holstein (2015) and "The Seduction of Agelessness, Take 2" by Molly Andrews (*Generations: Journal of the American Society on Aging*, Winter 2017–2018).

Audre Lorde's wonderfully political take on self-care comes from her book *A Burst of Light: And Other Essays*.

For a fascinating discussion about how stress-measuring instruments fall miserably short when it comes to measuring stress levels in midlife women, see "Undesirable Stressful Life Events, Impact, and Correlates During Midlife: Observations from the Seattle Midlife Women's Health Study" by Annette Joan Thomas, Ellen Sullivan Mitchell and Nancy Fugate Woods (*Women's Midlife Health*, January 2019). For a call for stress-measuring instruments that are more intersectional, see "Stress and Midlife Women's Health" by Lynnette Leidy Sievert, Nicole Jaff and Nancy Fugate Woods (*Women's Midlife Health*, March 16, 2018). And for a related discussion on how women are encouraged to treat stress as both an unavoidable fact of life and an issue that they somehow have to deal with on their own (as opposed to something requiring more structural, big-picture solutions), see *Connection, Compromise, and Control: Canadian Women Discuss Midlife* by Nancy Mandell, Susannah Wilson and Ann Duffy (2006).

The sources I consulted for the section of the chapter that deals with sleep include "Sleep Duration and Quality among Women Aged 40–59, by Menopausal Status" by Anjel Vahratian (National Center for Health Statistics, September 2017); "Sleep Disturbances in Midlife Women at the Cusp of the Menopausal Transition" by Holly J. Jones, Rochelle Zak and Kathryn A. Lee (*Journal of Clinical Sleep Medicine*, July 15, 2018); and "Chronic Stress Is Prospectively Associated with Sleep in Midlife Women: The SWAN Sleep Study" by Martica H. Hall et al. (*Sleep*, October 1, 2015).

The article about barriers to physical activity is "The Shaping of Midlife Women's Views of Health and Health Behaviors" by Kathleen Smith-DiJulio, Carol Windsor and Debra Anderson (*Qualitative Health Research*, July 2010).

For more about managing health-related worries and anxiety about aging, see "Multiple 'Old Ages': The Influence of Social

Context on Women's Aging Anxiety" by Anne E. Barrett and Erica L. Toothman (*The Journals of Gerontology: Series B*, November 2018) and *Shame and the Aging Woman: Confronting and Resisting Ageism in Contemporary Women's Writings* by J. Brooks Bouson (2018). For a related look at the health impacts of ageism, see "Longevity Increased by Positive Self-Perceptions of Aging" by Becca R. Levy, Martin D. Slade, Suzanne R. Kunkel and Stanislav V. Kasl (*Journal of Personality and Social Psychology*, August 2002).

For more about resisting both ageism and ableism and tapping into disability wisdom, I highly recommend *Brilliant Imperfection: Grappling with Cure* by Eli Clare (2017); *Care Work: Dreaming Disability Justice* by Leah Lakshmi Piepzna-Samarasinha (2018); *The Beginning of Everything: The Year I Lost My Mind and Found Myself* by Andrea J. Buchanan (2018); "Aging and Disability: Overcoming the 'Polite' Divide" by Susanne Schnell (*Generations: Journal of the American Society on Aging*, Winter 2017–2018); and "The Urgent Need for Disability Studies among Midlife Adults" by Carrie A. Karvonen-Gutierrez and Elsa S. Strotmeyer (*Women's Midlife Health*, August 2020).

Chapter 10: Body Love

Some of the books that I found helpful while I was researching this chapter were *Fit at Mid-Life: A Feminist Fitness Journey* by Samantha Brennan and Tracy Isaacs (2018); *The Body Is Not an Apology: The Power of Radical Self-Love* by Sonya Renee Taylor (2018); *The Seven Necessary Sins for Women and Girls* by Mona Eltahawy (2019); *Women Rowing North: Navigating Life's Currents and Flourishing as We Age* by Mary Pipher (2019); *Shame and the Aging Woman: Confronting and Resisting Ageism in Contemporary Women's Writings* by J. Brooks Bouson (2018); *Agewise: Fighting the New Ageism in*

America by Margaret Morganroth Gullette (2011); *In Our Prime: How Older Women Are Reinventing the Road Ahead* by Susan J. Douglas (2020); and *In Our Prime: The Invention of Middle Age* by Patricia Cohen (2012).

The Adrienne Rich quote about invisibility is cited in *Agewise: Fighting the New Ageism in America* by Margaret Morganroth Gullette (2011).

For more about "declining-attractiveness anxiety," see "Multiple 'Old Ages': The Influence of Social Context on Women's Aging Anxiety" by Anne E. Barrett and Erica L. Toothman (*The Journals of Gerontology: Series B*, November 2018).

For a fascinating discussion about how beauty is a product of culture, see "Women, Aging, and Beauty Culture: Navigating the Social Perils of Looking Old" by Laura Hurd Clarke (*Generations: Journal of the American Society on Aging*, Winter 2017-2018). Clarke notes that if we lived in a society that treated wrinkles and age spots as signs of beauty, we would all be rushing out to buy products that would help us look older, not younger. Her comment made me think of a really creative anti-ageism campaign that was conducted by the City of Toronto in November 2019. The campaign featured a fictitious product—aging cream: a cream that was supposed to *help you age more quickly*. The purpose of the campaign was to get people talking about aging and ageism. (The cream might have been fake but ageism definitely isn't.)

I was surprised to discover that there's a growing body of research on the subject of grey hair—a research trend that was actually kicked off in pre-pandemic times, incidentally. I actually came across an entire book that's been written on this issue: *Feminist Interrogations of Women's Head Hair: Crown of Glory and Shame*, edited by Sigal Barak-Brandes and Amit Kama (2018). One of the essays in the book ("Women's Grey Hair as an Abomination of the Body: Conceal and Pass, or Reveal and Subvert" by Vanessa Cecil, Louise F. Pendry, Jessica Salvatore and Tim Kurz) introduces the concept of "age-mediated aesthetic labour": the work people (mainly women) do to conceal evidence of age. And speaking of grey hair, the obnoxious piece of relationship advice that I cited in this chapter was drawn from Jane Haynes' article "How to Mentally Prepare for a Second Lockdown According to a Therapist" (British *Vogue*, September 30, 2020)—an article I read while I was celebrating the emergence of my own shimmering silver locks. (And, no, my marriage didn't end as a result of my decision to go grey.)

The two studies that I mentioned that focused on body image and weight were "Disordered Eating, Eating Disorders, and Body Image in Midlife and Older Women" by Karen L. Samuels, Margo M. Maine and Mary Tantillo (*Current Psychiatry Reports*, July 1, 2019) and "Understanding Body Image Dissatisfaction and Disordered Eating in Midlife Adults" by Sarah L. McGuinness and Joanne E. Taylor (*New Zealand Journal of Psychology*, April 1, 2016).

The statistics related to incontinence came from "Is Incontinence Associated with Menopause?" by Margaret Sherburn, Janet R. Guthrie, Emma C. Dudley, Helen E. O'Connell and Lorraine Dennerstein (*Obstetrics and Gynecology*, October 2001).

The resources I consulted while researching the sexuality section of the chapter include "Body Image, Attractiveness, and Sexual Satisfaction among Midlife Women: A Qualitative Study" by Holly N. Thomas, Megan Hamm, Sonya Borrero, Rachel Hess and Rebecca C. Thurston (*Journal of Women's Health*, January 2019); "Changes in Sexual Function among Midlife Women: 'I'm Older . . . and I'm Wiser'" by Holly N. Thomas, Megan Hamm, Rachel Hess and Rebecca C. Thurston (*Menopause*, March 2018); "Female Sexual Function at Midlife and Beyond" by Holly N. Thomas, Genevieve S. Neal-Perry and Rachel Hess (*Obstetrics and Gynecology Clinics of North America*,

December 2018); "Sexual Function among Women in Midlife: Findings from the Nurses' Health Study II" by Christiana von Hippel et al. (*Women's Health Issues*, July–August 2019); "All Shook Up: Sexuality of Mid- to Later Life Married Couples" by Amy C. Lodge and Debra Umberson (*Journal of Marriage and Family*, June 1, 2012); "Pain with Penetration" from the North American Menopause Society (article accessed in 2021); *There Are No Grown-ups: A Midlife Coming-of-Age Story* by Pamela Druckerman (2018); and a highly informative Twitter thread published by Sharron Hinchliff (@DrSharronH), who researches older adults' sexual and intimate relationships (published May 31, 2020).

Chapter 11: Midlife Epiphanies and Curveballs

Most of the material in this chapter was inspired by my interviews, but my thinking was also influenced by *Awakening at Midlife: A Guide to Reviving Your Spirit, Recreating Your Life, and Returning to Your Truest Self* by Kathleen A. Brehony (1997).

Chapter 12: A Little Help from My Friends

The following four articles were helpful to me in understanding and writing about midlife friendships: "A Life Span Developmental Perspective on Psychosocial Development in Midlife" by Tara L. Kuther and Kaitlyn Burnell (*Adultspan Journal*, April 2019); "Selfobject Experience in Long-Term Friendships of Midlife Women" by Michelle Piotrowski (*Psychoanalytic Social Work*, March 12, 2018); "The Role of Historical Change for Adult Development and Aging: Towards a Theoretical Framework about the How and the Why" by Johanna Drewelies, Oliver Huxhold and Denis Gerstorf (*Psychology and Aging*, December 2019); and "The Unsung Bonds of Friendship— and Caring—among Older Adults" by Brian de Vries (*Generations: Journal of the American Society on Aging*, Fall 2018).

Chapter 13: Family Matters

The following resources were most helpful to me in writing about both sandwich generation pressures and the unpaid and underpaid care work done by women: *"Time to Care: Unpaid and Underpaid Care Work and the Global Inequality Crisis: Summary"* (Oxfam International, January 2020); "Time Use: Total Work Burden, Unpaid Work, and Leisure" by Melissa Moyser and Amanda Burlock in *Women in Canada: A Gender-Based Statistical Report* (Statistics Canada, 2018); *The Care Manifesto: The Politics of Interdependence* by the Care Collective (2020); *The Care Crisis: What Caused It and How Can We End It?* by Emma Dowling (2021); *Who Cares? How to Reshape a Democratic Politics* by Joan C. Tronto (2015); *Women in Late Life: Critical Perspectives on Gender and Age* by Martha Holstein (2015); *This Chair Rocks: A Manifesto Against Ageism* by Ashton Applewhite (2015); and *In Our Prime: How Older Women Are Reinventing the Road Ahead* by Susan J. Douglas (2020).

For more on the time crunch faced by midlife parents, see "Time for Each Other: Work and Family Constraints among Couples" by Sarah M. Flood and Katie R. Genadek (*Journal of Marriage and Family*, February 2016). Flood and Genadek note that "parents share significantly less total and exclusive spousal time together than non-parents, although there is considerable variation among parents by age of the youngest child."

For more on midlife parenting, see "Millennials and Their Parents: Implications of the New Young Adulthood for

Midlife Adults" by Karen L. Fingerman (*Innovation in Aging*, November 2017); "A Family Affair: Family Typologies of Problems and Midlife Well-Being" by Karen L. Fingerman, Meng Huo, Jamie L. Graham, Kyungmin Kim and Kira S. Birditt (*Gerontologist*, November 3, 2018); "Only as Happy as the Least Happy Child: Multiple Grown Children's Problems and Successes and Middle-aged Parents' Well-being" by Karen L. Fingerman et al. (*The Journals of Gerontology: Series B*, March 2012); "Midlife in the 2020s: Opportunities and Challenges" by Frank J. Infurna, Denis Gerstorf and Margie E. Lachman (*American Psychologist*, May–June 2020); "Midlife Challenge or Welcome Departure? Cultural and Family-Related Expectations of Empty Nest Transitions" by Barbara A. Mitchell and Andrew V. Wister (*International Journal of Aging and Human Development*, December 2015); and "Reproductive Identity: An Emerging Concept" by Aurélie M. Athan (*American Psychologist*, May–June 2020).

For more about the joys and challenges of midlife couple relationships, see "Reclaiming the Second Phase of Life? Intersectionality, Empowerment and Respectability in Midlife Romance" by Sarah Milton and Kaveri Qureshi (*Sociological Research Online*, December 15, 2020); "The Role of Historical Change for Adult Development and Aging: Towards a Theoretical Framework about the How and the Why" by Johanna Drewelies, Oliver Huxhold and Denis Gerstorf (*Psychology and Aging*, December 2019); and *Couple Relationships in the Middle and Later Years: Their Nature, Complexity, and Role in Health and Illness*, edited by Jamila Bookwala (2016).

For more about being single at midlife and the tyranny of the so-called social clock, see "Starting 'Real' Life: Women Negotiating a Successful Midlife Single Identity" by Jennifer Moore and H. Lorraine Radtke (*Psychology of Women Quarterly*, March 2, 2015).

Chapter 14: Differently Political

The books that inspired a lot of the thinking for this chapter were *Unsettling Activisms: Critical Interventions on Aging, Gender, and Social Change*, edited by May Chazan, Melissa Baldwin and Patricia Evans (2018); *The Slow Moon Climbs: The Science, History, and Meaning of Menopause* by Susan P. Mattern (2019); *Flash Count Diary: Menopause and the Vindication of Natural Life* by Darcey Steinke (2019); *Mother Time: Women, Aging, and Ethics*, edited by Margaret Urban Walker (1999); *Women in Late Life: Critical Perspectives on Gender and Age* by Martha Holstein (2015); *In Our Prime: How Older Women Are Reinventing the Road Ahead* by Susan J. Douglas (2020); *Composing a Further Life: The Age of Active Wisdom* by Mary Catherine Bateson (2010); *Out of Time: The Pleasures and Perils of Ageing* by Lynne Segal (2013); *Radical Happiness: Moments of Collective Joy* by Lynne Segal (2017); *How to Do Nothing: Resisting the Attention Economy* by Jenny Odell (2019); *This Chair Rocks: A Manifesto Against Ageism* by Ashton Applewhite (2015); *Aging for Beginners* by Ezra Bayda with Elizabeth Hamilton (2018); *Becoming Wise: An Inquiry into the Mystery and Art of Living* by Krista Tippett (2016); *Out of the Wreckage: A New Politics for an Age of Crisis* by George Monbiot (2018); *Take Back the Fight: Organizing Feminism for the Digital Age* by Nora Loreto (2020); *One Long River of Song: Notes on Wonder* by Brian Doyle (2019); *Great Tide Rising: Towards Clarity and Moral Courage in a Time of Planetary Change* by Kathleen Dean Moore (2016); and *What Kind of Ancestor Do You Want to Be?* edited by John Hausdoerffer, Brooke Parry Hecht, Melissa K. Nelson and Katherine Kassouf Cummings (2021).

For more about how our time perspective flips at midlife, fuelling that sense of urgency that so many of us feel, see "The Bucket List Effect: Why Leisure Goals Are Often Deferred until Retirement" by Alexandra M. Freund (*American Psychologist*, May–June 2020). This study really helped me to understand why so many of the women I interviewed for this book kept circling around the same key phrase: "I'm running out of patience and time."

For more about the wisdom of older matriarchal elephants, see *The Slow Moon Climbs: The Science, History, and Meaning of Menopause* by Susan P. Mattern (2019). For a parallel discussion about whales, see *Flash Count Diary: Menopause and the Vindication of Natural Life* by Darcey Steinke (2019).

For more about the social determinants of health and Trish Hennessy's brilliant and important work in particular, visit the website for Think Upstream (thinkupstream.ca).

Paige's comment about the importance of living with questions as opposed to rushing to find answers made me think of something I read in Krista Tippett's book *Becoming Wise: An Inquiry into the Mystery and Art of Living* (2016). Tippett quoted some advice from the poet Rainer Maria Rilke, who emphasized the importance of living with questions as a means of living your way into the answer. I love that so much.

The quote from Kate Braestrup also appears in Tippett's book, but you should really track down the original May 2, 2016, conversation between the two women, which is archived on the website for the podcast and radio show *On Being*.

Leslie Jamison's essay "Lungs Full of Burning" appears in *Burn It Down: Women Writing about Anger*, edited by Lilly Dancyger (2019).

Conclusion: Midlife Reimagined

As I sat down to write the final pages of the book, I surrounded myself with the following books that touch on themes both personal and political: *Narrative Imagination and Everyday Life* by Molly Andrews (2013); *Composing a Further Life: The Age of Active Wisdom* by Mary

Catherine Bateson (2010); *In Our Prime: How Older Women Are Reinventing the Road Ahead* by Susan J. Douglas (2020); *Women in Late Life: Critical Perspectives on Gender and Age* by Martha Holstein (2015); *Connection, Compromise, and Control: Canadian Women Discuss Midlife* by Nancy Mandell, Susannah Wilson and Ann Duffy (2006); *Flash Count Diary: Menopause and the Vindication of Natural Life* by Darcey Steinke (2019); *Aging and Self-Realization: Cultural Narratives about Later Life* by Hanne Laceulle (2018); and "The Good Life and the Bad: Dialectics of Solidarity" by Shirin M. Rai (*Social Politics: International Studies in Gender, State and Society*, Spring 2018).

These books brought me comfort because they reminded me that so much of the change that I'm craving—that so many of us are craving—at this stage of our lives is for something much bigger than anything that can be tackled at the individual level. What we want more than anything else is to be given the gift of witnessing significant progress in our lifetimes—for things to be getting better, not worse. That's what I want for myself—and that's what I want for all of us. And if you've journeyed this far with me, I have to believe that that's what you want too. Thank you for making this journey with me—for daring to dream of better.

Permissions

Excerpts from *Narrative Imagination and Everyday Life* by Molly Andrews, copyright 2014. Reprinted by permission of Oxford University Press and reproduced with permission of the Licensor through PLSclear.

Excerpts from *This Chair Rocks: A Manifesto Against Ageism* by Ashton Applewhite, copyright 2016. Reprinted by permission of Celadon Books, a division of Macmillan Publishing.

Excerpts from *Composing a Further Life: The Age of Active Wisdom* by Mary Catherine Bateson, copyright 2010. Reprinted by permission of Penguin Random House.

Excerpts from *The Middlepause: Life after Youth* by Marina Benjamin, copyright 2016. Reprinted by permission of Scribe Publications.

Excerpts from *Awakening at Midlife: A Guide to Reviving Your Spirit, Recreating Your Life, and Returning to Your Truest Self* by Kathleen A. Brehony, copyright 1996. Reprinted by permission of Penguin Random House.

Excerpts from *Fit at Mid-Life: A Feminist Fitness Journey* by Samantha Brennan and Tracy Isaacs, copyright 2018. Reproduced with permission from Greystone Books.

Excerpts from *Unsettling Activisms: Critical Interventions on Aging, Gender, and Social Change* by May Chazan, Melissa Baldwin and Patricia Evans, copyright 2018. Reprinted by permission of Canadian Scholars.

Excerpts from *The Slow Moon Climbs: The Science, History, and Meaning of Menopause* by Susan P. Mattern, copyright 2019. Reprinted by permission of Princeton University Press.

Excerpt from *How to Do Nothing: Resisting the Attention Economy* by Jenny Odell, copyright 2019. Reprinted by permission of Melville House.

Excerpt from "The Life Narrative at Midlife" by Dan P. McAdams in *Rereading Personal Narrative and Life Course: New Directions for Child and Adolescent Development* edited by B. Schiff, copyright 2014. Used by permission of John Wiley and Sons.

Excerpts from *Flash Count Diary: Menopause and the Vindication of Natural Life* by Darcey Steinke, copyright 2016. Reprinted by permission of Sarah Crichton Books, a division of Farrar, Straus and Giroux.

Excerpt from "Virtues and Age" by Sara Ruddick, in *Mother Time: Women, Aging, and Ethics* by Margaret Urban Walker, copyright 1999. All rights reserved. Reprinted by permission of Rowman & Littlefield.

Excerpts from *The Body Is Not an Apology: The Power of Radical Self-Love* by Sonya Renee Taylor, copyright 2021. Reprinted by permission of Berrett-Koehler Publishers Inc.

Excerpt from *Becoming Wise: An Inquiry into the Mystery and Art of Living* by Krista Tippett, copyright 2016. Reprinted by permission of Penguin Random House.

Index

About the Author

For decades, Ann Douglas was Canada's go-to expert on all things parenting. Now she's turning her attention to the glorious messiness that is midlife. She is the author of twenty-five non-fiction books, including many best-selling titles in the parenting category, and a passionate and inspiring speaker who delivers keynote addresses and leads small-group workshops at conferences and online events. Ann and her husband, Neil, live on a lake in rural Ontario, where she is hard at work on her first novel.

Twitter: @anndouglas
Instagram: @AnnMDouglas
Facebook: @NavigatingTheMessyMiddle, @TheMotherofAllBooks
Website: anndouglas.ca